A Good Night's Sleep

Simple, Effective Ways to Overcome Insomnia

BARBARA WEXLER, MPH

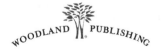

WOODLAND PUBLISHING

For permissions, ordering information, or bulk quantity discounts, contact: Woodland Publishing, Salt Lake City, UT

Visit our Web site: www.woodlandpublishing.com
Toll-free number (800) 777-BOOK

Note: The information in this book is for educational purposes only and is not recommended as a means of diagnosing or treating an illness. All matters concerning physical and mental health should be supervised by a health practitioner knowledgeable in treating that particular condition. Neither the publisher nor the authors directly or indirectly dispense medical advice, nor do they prescribe any remedies or assume any responsibility for those who choose to treat themselves.

ISBN 978-1-58054-102-2

Printed in the United States of America

Contents

Understanding Sleep

All men whilst they are awake are in one common world: but each of them, when he is asleep, is in a world of his own.

—Plutarch

We spend a nearly a third of our lives sleeping, and while we know that sleep is necessary, its precise role in our lives has not yet been identified. In fact, the function of sleep is one of the most persistent and perplexing mysteries in life science.

Still, we understand some of the changes that occur in the body during sleep and how these changes affect our health and our lives. Since we devote so much of our lives to sleep, and because so many of us—about one-quarter of Americans—suffer from sleep problems, let's take a closer look at what happens during sleep, what causes us to sleep, and how our bodies respond to both sleep and sleep deprivation.

Sleep Is Not Optional—It's Essential

It's hard to convince children who want to stay up all night rather than miss a moment of fun that sleep is not waste of valuable time. Sleep is not optional—it's essential. It is not only necessary for all of our physiological functions, including motor activity and cognition (thinking, reasoning, intuition and perception), but also for our very survival. Animal studies have repeatedly demonstrated that when deprived of sleep, laboratory animals die in a matter of weeks, in much the same way that they would if they were denied food.

Sleep appears to be even more important for the brain than it is for the body. Sleep is thought to influence cognition in many ways. Scientists believe that it helps eliminate one or more toxic by-products of wakefulness, or restores and replenishes neural substrates (the substances on which enzymes act) needed for optimal mental function.

Recent research reveals that sleep actually reorganizes brain connections to improve performance. Sleep helps to strengthen memories and improve physical performance by producing large-scale changes in brain activity that makes a skill less dependent on conscious thought. Consider this a tangible example of this function of sleep:

Harvard Medical School researchers taught college students a simple finger-tapping task and then retested them at the task twelve hours later, after a full night's sleep or twelve daytime hours without sleep. The researchers monitored the participants' brain activity using magnetic resonance imaging (MRI is a noninvasive procedure that produces a two-dimensional view of the organs it scans).

Subjects who slept performed the task with fewer errors than those in the daytime test group and showed greater brain activation in the parts of the brain that control speed and accuracy as well as the areas that help to create memory. This increased activation suggests that sleep reinforced the memory of the task in motor-control areas of the brain, enabling the subjects to perform the task more quickly and accurately. Furthermore, subjects who slept showed decreased brain activity in the areas of the brain involved in conscious monitoring of physical movement and in several emotion-regulating regions, suggesting that as memory of the task was reinforced, the task became easier to perform without thinking about it too much. This, in turn, may have reduced the emotional workload involved in performing the task.

The researchers assert that more research is needed to determine whether a full night's sleep prompts these changes in the brain, or whether they are prompted by a specific stage of sleep. These findings are not only important in terms of learning skills, such as playing a musical instrument or a sport, but also for post-injury or illness rehabilitation and for examining the relationship between sleep disturbances and learning problems.

Why Do We Sleep?

> *Sleeping is no mean art: for its sake one must stay awake all day.*
> —Friedrich Nietzsche

Many theories have been proposed to explain why we sleep, but most account for only one aspect of our need for sleep or our sleep behavior. One hypothesis posits that sleep is simply a period for rest and recovery, during which we replenish the energy we've expended during waking hours. This hypothesis is supported by the fact that the brain remains active during sleep, presumably to direct the restoration process. However, there is scant evidence that physical repair occurs more rapidly or more frequently during sleep than it does during periods of rest or relaxation. For example, protein synthesis, which is vital for repair, declines during sleep, at least in part because we are not supplying the body with the nutrients it needs to perform this task, since we essentially fast during sleep.

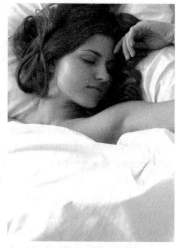

A peaceful night's sleep

Another theory proposes that sleep conserves energy and other biological resources in the body and that total sleep time is proportional to the amount of energy expended during wakefulness. This theory is supported by the fact that species with longer durations of sleep have higher core body temperatures and higher metabolic rates, and by the observation that metabolic rates drop when we fall asleep and remain low throughout sleep. This theory also partly explains why we feel so sleepy when we're sick or battling bacterial or viral infections—sleep enables the body to conserve energy and other resources, which may then be used to fend off infection.

Still other theories assert that REM sleep (the stage of sleep characterized by rapid eye movement), high levels of brain activity, and dreams, is necessary for brain development, discharge of emotions, and stress relief. Some sleep researchers contend that activity in the regions of the brain that control emotions, decisionmaking, and complex social interactions is reduced during sleep to enable us to recharge so that when we're awake, we perform these functions of daily living more effectively.

So while the purpose of sleep has not yet been fully determined, there is some evidence that it is important for selectively integrating and reinforcing learning and memories. This theory, called memory consolidation, proposes that during the course of a typical day we learn and experience many things—only some of which are important to remember. Conceivably, when we sleep, our experiences and the information we've received during the day may be sorted and prioritized, allowing some to be discarded and others to be imprinted in our minds.

Research reveals that people who get a good night's sleep are faster learners and perform better on tests requiring spatial perception, eye-hand coordination, and memory. People who are chronically sleep deprived have shorter attention spans, longer reaction times, and have compromised cognitive function overall. This research confirms practically everyone's experience—when we don't get enough sleep, our thinking is slower, we're less able to concentrate on the tasks at hand, and we just don't feel as sharp as we do when we're well rested.

Recently, researchers at the University of California and Stanford University demonstrated that sleep deprivation impairs spatial learning. Learning spatial tasks increases the production of cells in the hippocampus—the part of the brain involved with spatial memory. Apparently, sleep plays an important role in helping these new brain cells to survive. The researchers also posited that sleep deprivation essentially undoes the rejuvenating effects of learning on the brain.

The Biology of Sleep

A common misconception about sleep is that it's a quiet process during which the brain and body slow down or shut down in order to rest. And while it is true that there is a slight decline in metabolic rate during sleep, none of the organs or physiological processes in the body shuts down when we sleep.

Sleep is an active, dynamic, complex, and highly regulated activity characterized by ever-changing levels of consciousness. During sleep, some systems perform specific tasks. For example, the endocrine system increases production of hormones, including growth hormone and prolactin. The pituitary gland secretes human growth hormone during sleep, especially in children and adolescents; this probably explains why parents tell their reluctant-to-retire offspring that they need to sleep in order to grow. The release of human growth hormone during sleep is likely involved with some of the repair processes that occur during sleep.

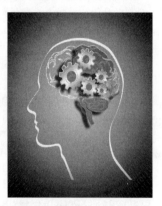

Many neurological processes are involved in sleep.

Other hormones are secreted into the blood during sleep, including follicle stimulating hormone (FSH) and luteinizing hormone (LH), which play pivotal roles in growth and reproduction. Many sleep researchers contend that the sleep-dependent release of LH is the signal event that initiates the onset of sexual maturation and puberty.

Similarly, there are periods of heightened brain activity during sleep. Though we're less sensitive to stimulation (such as sound, light, and touch) than we are when we're awake, our brain activity is more varied than it is during waking hours. Delta waves, which indicate deep, slow brain activity, increase during deep, dreamless sleep. They are measured using an encephalogram (also known as an EEG, which graphically records the electrical activity of the brain) and occur with high voltage and low frequency.

Along with a somewhat slower metabolism and complex, active brainwave patterns, our bodies assume relaxed positions, largely because we are usually lying down and making less use of our skeletal muscles. When we are awake, these muscles must work to support our postures, even when we are sitting quietly or are otherwise inactive. Still, our bodies do move frequently while we sleep.

THE CIRCADIAN RHYTHM IS OUR INTERNAL BIOLOGICAL CLOCK

> *It's a cruel season that makes you get ready for bed while it's light out.*
> —John Calvin

Biological clocks are genetically programmed physiological systems that enable us and other animals to live in harmony with natural patterns, such as the rising and setting of the sun and the changing seasons. Our internal biological clocks regulate when we sleep, generally causing us to feel awake during the day and sleepy at night. These biological clocks operate in a pattern known as a circadian rhythm (from the Latin *circa*, which means "about," and *diem*, which means "day"). Circadian rhythms are regularly recurring changes in physiological and mental processes that occur over the course of a day. They help to coordinate the timing of our internal bodily functions, including sleep and our interactions with the external world.

In humans and other mammals, circadian rhythms are governed by light and dark. The circadian clock in mammals is located in the suprachiasmatic nucleus (SCN), a brain structure located in the hypothalamus, just above the point where the optic nerve crosses. Light reaches photoreceptors in the retina—tissue at the back of the eye—and generates signals that travel along the optic nerve to the SCN.

These signals go to several brain regions, including the pineal gland, which responds to light-induced signals by switching off production of the hormone melatonin. The body's level of melatonin typically rises when darkness falls, prompting us to feel sleepy. The SCN also governs functions such as body temperature, hormone secretion, urine production, and changes in blood pressure that are synchronized with the circadian rhythm. When cells in the SCN are destroyed, the affected animal loses its regular sleep/wake rhythm.

Proteins called cryptochromes, which are present throughout the body, are also involved in perceiving changes in light and setting the body's clock.

Since the circadian clock in humans has a natural day length of slightly more than twenty-four hours, the clock must be reset to match the day length. Although circadian rhythms are primarily governed by light and darkness, they may be affected by nearly any kind of time cue, such as the ringing of church

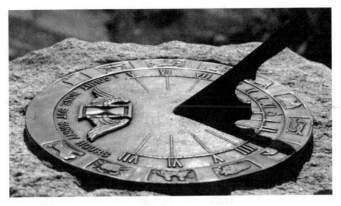

A sundial: ancient way to measure time

bells, the buzz of an alarm clock, the rattle of a garbage truck, the unrelenting drone of a car alarm, or the timing of meals. Such outside influences that affect circadian rhythm are known as *zeitgebers* (German for "time givers").

These influences are so powerful and pervasive that even in the absence of environmental time cues, circadian rhythms persist with a period close to twenty-four hours. Research reveals that even when people are kept in temporal isolation— without clocks, changes in sunlight, or other cues to tell them whether it's night or day or how much time has passed—their internal circadian clocks have a period (also known as tau) of slightly longer than twenty-four hours. This tau is also observed in many blind people.

Even short-term disruption of the circadian rhythm can be quite uncomfortable. For example, travelers often experience jet lag when travel involves changing time zones because their zeitgebers occur at new times, shaking up the circadian rhythm. Symptoms of jet lag may include feeling groggy and fatigued, or suffering from depression, headaches, altered appetite and sleeping problems. It usually takes several days for the body's cycles to adjust to a new time zone.

And if you thought that teenagers stayed up late and slept in simply because they wanted to party all night long, you'll be surprised to learn that researchers have found that adolescents experience a delay in the circadian timing system that results in a tendency for them to stay up later and sleep in later. In response to this finding, some educators have suggested that the optimal start time for high schools might be mid-morning instead of eight or nine o'clock. No doubt, sleepy teens would concur with this proposed change!

Disruption of circadian rhythms not only affects sleep, energy, and concentration, but also has been shown to trigger mania (excessively intense enthusiasm, interest, or desire) in people who suffer from bipolar disorder (also known as manic depression). Other diseases and disorders are affected by circadian rhythms, too. Heart attacks occur more frequently in the morning, while asthma attacks occur more often at night.

The Sleep Cycle

Sleep is a cyclical process, and while sleep/wake cycles vary from person to person, sleepiness and sleep recur in regular, rhythmic patterns. There are two strikingly different types of sleep—rapid eye movement (REM) sleep, which is when we dream, and non-rapid eye movement (NREM) sleep.

NREM sleep is divided into four stages that correspond to the amplitude and frequency of brain-wave activity that occurs during each stage.

Stage 1 is very light sleep, not unlike very deep relaxation. When we are relaxed but still awake, our brain waves become slower, increase in amplitude, and move in regular, synchronous phases. These types of waves are called alpha waves and are often associated with states of deep relaxation like those achieved in meditation and biofeedback.

During stage 1, an EEG shows theta waves, which have a higher amplitude and lower frequency than alpha waves. Eye movements slow, as does muscle activity. Stage 1 sleep, sometimes called drowsiness, is a brief transition from wakefulness and usually lasts just five to ten minutes. It's really easy to awaken someone in stage 1 sleep.

In stage 2, theta waves continue and are joined by two

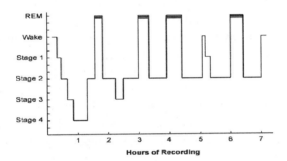

Sleep stages over a seven-hour period

unusual brain waves called sleep spindles (sudden increases in wave frequency and K complexes), which are sudden increases in wave amplitude. During stage 2, eye movements steadily slow and then stop, heart rate slows and body temperature decreases. Stage 2 is also a relatively light stage of sleep. In fact, when people wake someone from stage 1 or 2 sleep, they may deny that they were sleeping at all.

Stages 3 and 4 are deep sleep states, known as slow-wave, or delta, sleep. In these stages and during the transition from stage 3 to 4, there are increasingly more slow brain waves that occur with rhythmic continuity. The muscle activity of sleep is low, but the muscles retain their ability to function. Eye movements normally don't occur during these stages of sleep, except for very slow eye movements, usually at the beginning of stage 3. In stage 4, it is extremely hard to be awakened by external stimuli. It's also the easiest stage from which to return to sleep should you be awakened. It's during stage 4 that some sleepers seemingly mindlessly turn off their alarm clocks and immediately return to sleep.

Sleep begins with NREM and then cycles through REM and NREM in 90 to 120 minute sessions, with each stage lasting from five to fifteen minutes. This pattern is called an ultradian rhythm because it is a cycle that repeats more than once every twenty-four hours. (In contrast, a circadian rhythm is based on twenty-four-hour intervals.)

The NREM-REM cycle repeats itself from four to six times each night, but as the night wears on the amount of deep NREM sleep decreases and the amount of REM sleep increases. A typical sleep pattern doubles back to repeat stages 2 and 3 before REM sleep begins, so it looks something like this:

Relaxed wakefulness
↓
Stage 1
↓
Stage 2
↓
Stage 3
↓
Stage 4
↓
Stage 3
↓
Stage 2
↓
REM sleep (about 100 minutes into the sleep cycle)

RAPID EYE MOVEMENT SLEEP

Rapid eye movement (REM) sleep is also known as stage 5, or paradoxical, sleep, because during REM sleep two seemingly opposite actions occur—the brain increases activity and excitement, and a kind of muscular paralysis occurs that is thought to prevent us from physically acting out our dreams. REM sleep is easily distinguished from NREM sleep by cerebral and physiological changes, especially its characteristic rapid eye movements, which likely occur when we "watch" our dreams as we might watch a movie. Although the brain-wave patterns observed in REM sleep appear similar to those seen during stage 1 sleep, the physiological similarities between REM and NREM sleep end there.

For example, during NREM sleep the heart rate slows, while in REM sleep it increases and varies. Similarly, blood pressure decreases during NREM sleep while it increases by as much as 30 percent during REM sleep. Blood flow to the brain during NREM sleep is comparable to blood flow during wakefulness, but it increases by anywhere from 50 to 200 percent during REM sleep, depending on the region of the brain. Breathing also slows during NREM sleep and increases during REM sleep. Interestingly, while coughing is suppressed during REM sleep, brief periods (during which breathing stops, called sleep apnea) are more likely to occur.

Even our body's thermostat responds differently during NREM and REM sleep. During NREM sleep, body temperature stabilizes at a lower set point than when we're awake, which means that shivering—the body's reflexive response to cold that aims to create warmth by expending energy—begins at lower temperatures than it would when we are awake. Also, while we rarely are sexually aroused during NREM sleep, both men and women are more likely to become aroused during REM sleep.

The first period of REM sleep generally lasts about ten minutes, and each recurring REM stage lasts a little longer, with the final one in the sleep cycle lasting an hour. It is pretty common to wake briefly at the end of a REM phase. Typically, adults get about 90 to 120 minutes of REM sleep per night, which constitutes about 20 percent of their sleep. The proportion of time spent in REM sleep varies with age—newborn babies spend more than 80 percent of their total sleep time in REM, while adults over age seventy spend less than 10 percent of sleep time in REM sleep.

MEASURING REM SLEEP

Polysomnography simultaneously records the three measures that define the main stages of sleep and wakefulness. Where an EEG offers information about electrical activity from one area of the brain, muscle tone may be measured with an electromyogram (EMG), and eye movements during sleep are recorded using an electrooculogram (EOG). EEG readings distinguish the various stages of sleep, while the EMG and EOG distinguish REM sleep from NREM sleep.

An EEG recorded during REM sleep reveals fast, desynchronized activity that appears random when compared with an

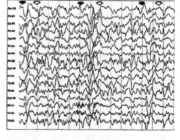

EEG taken during REM sleep

EEG recorded during NREM sleep. An EEG recorded during REM sleep resembles an EEG recorded during wakefulness—low voltage with a faster mix of frequencies.

REM sleep features bursts of rapid eye movements. The eyes are not constantly moving, but they dart back and forth or up and down. They also stop for a while and then jerk back and forth again. Always, like waking eye movements, both eyes move together in the same direction. Although the muscles that move our bodies are quiet during REM sleep, which essentially paralyzes us, other muscles (such as the heart, lungs, and diaphragm) and blood vessels function as they would in waking hours.

The Chemistry of Sleep and Wakefulness

Neurotransmitters, naturally occurring chemicals in the brain that transmit messages from one nerve cell to another, are involved in sleep and wakefulness. Neurons in the brain stem, which connects the brain with the spinal cord, produce neurotransmitters such as serotonin and norepinephrine, which keep parts of the brain active while we are awake. Other neurons at the base of the brain begin signaling when we fall asleep. These neurons also act to dampen or turn off the signals that keep us awake.

Research suggests that adenosine, a sleep-producing substance, accumulates in certain areas of the brain and in our blood while we are awake and causes drowsiness. Adenosine is a breakdown product of adenosine triphosphate (ATP), which is an important energy reserve in cells. While we sleep, adenosine gradually breaks down. Research studies using animals have found that adenosine levels in the brain rise during sleep deprivation and return to baseline during sleep. The caffeine in your eye-opening morning cup of coffee is thought to promote wakefulness by blocking adenosine receptors. Other substances thought to promote sleep are proinflammatory cytokines (interleukin-1), prostaglandin D, and growth-hormone-releasing hormone.

The most important part of the brain in regulating sleep duration is the hypothalamus. The role of the hypothalamus was recognized after the worldwide spread of encephalitis lethargica in the early twentieth century. Thought to be a viral infection, encephalitis lethargica caused severe sleep disturbances in infected people. Most patients became profoundly sleepy, but others suffered from insomnia. The patients afflicted with sleepiness were found to have lesions in the posterior hypothalamus, while those with insomnia had lesions in the anterior hypothalamus.

The anterior hypothalamus contains groups of hypothalamic neurons that produce the neurotransmitter gamma-aminobutyric acid (GABA). Projections of these GABA neurotransmitters inhibit the firing of cells involved in wakefulness. Several groups of neurons are inhibited by this action—including neurons containing histamine, norepinephrine, serotonin, hypocretin, and glutamate—and this inhibition promotes sleep. Antihistamines are known to produce sedation and sleepiness because histamine plays a key role in maintaining wakefulness. Histaminergic neurons fire most rapidly in the wakeful state and turn off during REM sleep.

Hypocretin (also called orexin) was discovered in 1998, and its role in sleep was identified in 2001. The concentration of the hypocretin-producing neurons in the hypothalamus is highest during wakefulness. Hypocretin levels also increase during periods of forced sleep deprivation. Other undiscovered transmitters are undoubtedly involved in maintaining wakefulness and promoting sleep.

The Miracle of Sleep

For fast-acting relief, try slowing down.
—Lily Tomlin

If it's not a problem in our lives, we tend to take sleep for granted. But poor sleep patterns can create a host of problems. People who don't get enough sleep, or whose sleep is not refreshing, are frequently at risk of experiencing episodes of microsleep—moments of falling asleep that they may not even remember. Obviously, these episodes can be extremely dangerous, especially if they occur while driving or during other such activities.

Sleep is a time when the body regenerates and detoxifies. When sleep is disturbed, it sets the stage for problems ranging from accelerated aging, disruptive variations in mood and attention, and the potential for increased susceptibility to infections and other immune system problems.

Every night, when we enter REM sleep, we dream. Everyone dreams, whether or not they consciously remember their dreams. As we discussed, some neurologists and sleep researchers believe that REM sleep is an essential period in which the brain reorganizes memory and experience.

We know from sleep deprivation experiments that people who are continually blocked from entering REM sleep undergo rapid mental deterioration. Within a few days, they may even start to exhibit signs of severe mental disorders like auditory and visual hallucinations, disordered thinking, paranoia, and psychotic delusions. In an otherwise healthy person, these symptoms are temporary and quickly regress when REM sleep is once again permitted.

When sleep suffers, affected individuals may begin to exhibit signs of sleep deprivation, which can place tremendous strain on work, personal relationships, and self-esteem. Unfortunately, the degradation of sleep is a vicious cycle. Stress or other causes of sleep disorders interfere with falling asleep or obtaining adequate sleep. This lack of sleep in turn creates more symptoms of stress. And the impact of this spiraling problem, through its effects on mood, attention, and cognitive function can cause problems that may become new sources of stress. The importance of restful sleep simply can't be overstated.

How Much Sleep Do We Need?

In general, small animals need more sleep than larger ones. For example, brown bats sleep nearly twenty hours a day, and owl monkeys sleep seventeen hours. Human infants, sleep sixteen hours (though many exhausted parents wish that eight of those hours would be at night, consecutive, and uninterrupted). Most human adolescents need a minimum of nine hours of sleep—roughly the same amount as chimpanzees (9.7 hours), baboons (10.3 hours), and bottle-nosed dolphins (10.4 hours).

Adult humans need about eight hours of sleep, comparable to pigs (7.8 hours) and much more than cows (3.9 hours), horses (2.9 hours), or giraffes (1.9 hours). Age is the strongest factor that affects how much sleep we need, as well as the continuity of our sleep and the distribution of sleep stages through the night. The sleep patterns of newborn infants are dramatically different from those of adults.

Newborns and infants sleep twice as much as adults do, and they enter sleep through REM. During the first year of life, REM sleep is a full 50 percent of total sleep time; it decreases to adult levels—20 to 25 percent—by age three, where it remains until old age. Slow-wave sleep isn't present at birth, but it develops by about two to six months. The amount of slow-wave sleep peaks in childhood and then steadily declines such that it's nearly nonexistent in older adults.

Along with the loss of slow-wave sleep, older adults also have more fragile and fragmented sleep, more stage 1 sleep. They are less likely to be able to sleep continuously at night and remain continuously wakeful during the day. About half of all people over sixty-five have frequent sleeping problems, such as insomnia, and deep sleep stages in many older adults often become very short or stop completely.

Contrary to popular belief, the need for sleep does not diminish with advancing age; the ability to maintain sleep does—older people don't *need* less sleep, they just *get* less sleep. It's not yet known whether changes such as becoming more sensitive to light and noise are normal parts of healthy aging or result from chronic health problems or chronic pain or even the treatment for these problems.

The amount of sleep we need is the amount that enables us to feel alert and refreshed and avoid feeling sleepy or falling asleep unintentionally during the day. For most young adults, this is between seven and eight hours per night, but it varies from person to person depending on their circumstances. Some people claim to function well on as few as five hours of sleep per night, and others report that they need ten hours per night in order to feel well rested. Women in the first trimester of pregnancy often need more sleep than usual. Genetics also play some part in determining the amount of sleep needed.

Daytime sleepiness is the simplest indicator of inadequate sleep. If you feel drowsy during the day, even during a boring meeting or class, then you haven't had enough sleep. If you routinely fall asleep as soon as your head hits the pillow— within minutes of lying down, then you might suffer from sleep deprivation and possibly even a sleep disorder. Microsleeps— very brief episodes of sleep in an otherwise awake person—are another mark of sleep deprivation. Often people are entirely unaware that they are succumbing to microsleeps. The frenetic pace and increased time demands of Western industrialized societies have caused so much sleep deprivation that we've become accustomed to feeling sleepy rather than well rested.

When our sleep needs are not met, we incur a progressive sleep debt, and eventually the body requires that the debt be paid in full. Even though we may become accustomed to feeling sleepy during waking hours, we appear unable to adapt to getting less sleep than our bodies require.

How Much Sleep Do We Get?

The short answer is that many Americans just don't get enough sleep. The National Sleep Foundation (NSF) conducts a biannual survey of Americans' sleep habits and patterns. The 2005 survey considered the sleep patterns and problems of men and women, the 2006 survey looked at adolescents' sleep patterns, and the 2007 poll focused on the sleep habits of American women.

The NSF 2005 survey found that 75 percent of American adults experience symptoms of a sleep problem at least a few nights per week and that American adults slept an average of 6.9 hours per night (6.8 hours a night on weekdays and 7.4 hours a night on weekends). Forty percent of survey respondents said they got less than seven hours of sleep on weekdays. From 2001 to 2005, a decreasing proportion of respondents—38 percent in 2001 and 26 percent in 2005—said they slept eight or more hours per night on weekdays. Just one-half of the respondents (49 percent) reported getting "a good night's sleep" every night or nearly every night.

The 2006 survey revealed that (20 percent) of adolescents get the recommended nine hours of sleep on school nights, and 45 percent of teens sleep less than eight hours on school nights.

Inadequate sleep has an impact on nearly every aspect of teens' lives. The survey reported the following:

- At least once a week more than 28 percent of high school students fall asleep in school, 22 percent fall asleep doing homework, and 14 percent arrive late or miss school because they oversleep.

- Teens who get insufficient amounts of sleep are more likely than their peers to have lower grades, while 80 percent of

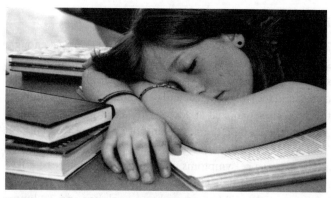

Many teens don't get adequate sleep at night.

adolescents who get an optimal amount of sleep reported earning As and Bs in school. More than one-half (51 percent) of adolescent drivers had driven while drowsy during the previous year, and 15 percent of drivers in tenth to twelfth grades drive while drowsy at least once a week.

- Among teens who described themselves as unhappy, tense, and nervous, 73 percent report that they don't get enough sleep at night, and 59 percent are excessively sleepy during the day.

- More than one-quarter (28 percent) of adolescents say they're too tired to exercise.

- The amount of sleep adolescents get declines as they get older—sixth graders slept an average of 8.4 hours on school nights, while twelfth graders slept just 6.9 hours.

The 2007 Sleep in America Poll painted a picture of American women as continually sleep deprived due to caring for young children, conditions such as pregnancy and menopause, work or family stress, or because of pets. Survey participants reported that lack of sleep caused them to be late to work, suffer high stress, feel depressed or anxious, skip their usual exercise routines, feel too tired for sex, drive while drowsy, and have little or no time for personal and family relationships.

Working mothers, whom the study termed the "briefcase and backpack" group, seemed to be the most affected. Their Herculean efforts to manage full-time work schedules while juggling family responsibilities left them staying up late and skimping on sleep so often that they were continually sleep deprived.

The analysis of the survey data concluded that the primary cause of sleep deprivation was women's efforts to fulfill their responsibilities: professional work, childcare, family needs, and relationships with their husbands and close friends.

Other key findings from the 2007 survey are as follows:

- Sleep and exercise are the first things women sacrifice when they have too much to do.

- Nearly half of all women say they don't get enough sleep every night.

- Thirty percent of pregnant women and 42 percent of women with newborns report rarely getting a good night's sleep, while 84 percent suffer from insomnia a few nights per week.

- Women wake frequently during the night in response to noise (39 percent), the need to care for children (20 percent), and the need to care for pets (17 percent).

- Forty-seven percent of women say they have no one to help with childcare at night.

- Thirty-five percent of working moms admit that they drove while drowsy.

- Sixty-five percent of women use caffeinated beverages to cope with the lack of sleep.

Dreams: The Royal Road to the Unconscious

Our truest life is when we are in our dreams awake.

—Henry David Thoreau

The Eye of the Needle

Elias Howe was a man on a mission. By the mid-1840s, after spending years on a quest to invent a truly practical sewing machine, his money and his patience were nearly at an end. His wife took in odd sewing jobs to pay their bills and maintain their modest New England home. But as simple as the task of designing a sewing machine first appeared, it resisted the best efforts not only of Howe but of all the greatest inventors of the day.

One night, Howe had a frightening dream. He found himself chased through the jungle by a band of wild savages. After herding the hapless inventor into a stewpot, the savages circled around, menacing him with their spears. Through his terror at their wild thrusting, Howe suddenly noticed something so odd and out of place that it momentarily drove the fear from his mind. Looking carefully at the spears, he noticed that each one had a hole in the tip. Howe awakened and found himself consumed by this one strange detail.

Suddenly, the meaning became clear. In a regular sewing needle—the kind that had been used since time immemorial—the hole was always placed at the far end, the last part of the needle to be drawn through the cloth. It was such a basic fact that no one had ever questioned it. But Howe realized in a flash of dream-inspired insight that by putting the hole at the opposite end—in the tip, just as he'd seen it in the natives' spears—he could easily pierce the cloth and create a locking stitch from below. In the dreaming state, Howe's mind was able to circumvent the deeply ingrained habits of convention and reveal a simple idea that quite literally changed the world in which we live.

A Universal Experience

> *Why does no one confess his sins? Because he is yet in them. It is for a man who has awoke from sleep to tell his dreams.*
>
>   —Seneca

Scientists who study sleep tell us that everyone dreams, whether we consciously remember our dreams or not. They know this because during the dreaming state certain parts of the brain and nervous system show consistent patterns of activity that resemble many aspects of the waking state. These patterns are, in turn, very different from the activity that is measured during other phases of the sleep experience.

During an average night's sleep, we usually dream for more than two hours, and most dreaming occurs during REM sleep. While reports of dreaming are most frequent and vivid when an individual is woken from REM sleep, dreams do occur at the beginning of sleep as well as during NREM sleep.

How universal is dreaming? Recently, Massachusetts Institute of Technology researchers Drs. Matthew Wilson and Kenway Louie demonstrated that rats appear to dream while they sleep. They implanted microsensors in the rats' brains that detected patterns of electrical activity during sleep that precisely matched those found during specific activities, such as running through a maze. The realization that dreaming is not a uniquely human activity may cause us to shift our understanding of the nature and origin of the dream state.

Before exploring various theories of why we dream, it's interesting to note that many traditions, from ancient times to the present day, have used the insights, information, and feelings associated with dreams in conscious and positive ways. Dreaming has sometimes been compared to looking through a kaleidoscope. It really doesn't matter what's inside the kaleidoscope—shells, pebbles, bits of shattered glass, broken watch parts. That's because the kaleidoscope imposes symmetry on whatever it contains. It creates something beautiful, regardless of the input. The human mind does the same thing, constantly building connections and searching for meaning. Therefore even if, as some researchers believe, the process of dreaming begins with random thoughts and feelings, they can be organized by our sleeping mind into wonderfully non-random patterns.

Many dream work traditions, from the Native American Hopis to contemporary "dream groups" like those organized by noted dream work pioneer Reverend Jeremy Taylor, realize that making the effort to consciously remember and work with our dreams can, in turn, alter and even enhance the dreaming experience. Seasoned dream workers find that they can even "incubate" their dreams to focus on a particular emotional, physical, intellectual, or spiritual challenge, consciously carrying the concerns of the day into the shadowy, creative processes of the night. It seems that the intention of seeking meaning in our dreams may actually help build more robust bridges between our everyday waking awareness and the information available to us in the dreaming state.

SEEDS OF CHANGE

Peace, peace! he is not dead, he doth not sleep
He hath awakened from the dream of life—

—Percy Bysshe Shelley

For many years, Reverend Jeremy Taylor has conducted groups for people who wish to explore their dreams. He has written several books about dream work, including *Dream Work: Techniques for Discovering the Creative Power in Dreams* (Paulist Press, 1982) and *Where People Fly and Water Runs Uphill: Using Dreams to Tap the Wisdom of the Unconscious* (Warner Books, 1993). He has conducted numerous dream groups in schools, hospices, prisons—anywhere people have expressed an interest in coming together to work creatively with the aspects of their consciousness experienced in the dream state. Unlike the more familiar discipline of dream analysis, his process is not a search to impose meaning onto the dream from the outside but rather, to create a living laboratory in which each person has the chance to discover both the uniquely personal and the archetypal dimensions their dreams may contain.

A number of years ago, the members of an ongoing dream group noticed that one member came to the session every week, offered helpful insights into other people's dreams, but had never shared a dream of his own. The members of the group encouraged him to share with them from his own experience. However, he demurred, telling them that he "never dreamed."

The group was not dissuaded. "Everyone dreams," they said, and encouraged him to dredge up something, however insignificant and fragmentary it might at first seem, as a starting point for their shared process. The young man reflected for a few moments and said, "OK. The only thing I can remember is a sense of pastel colors. That's all."

Once he'd shared this small detail the man was embarrassed. "That's not a lot to go on," he admitted and offered to give up his place so that someone else could share a bigger, more important dream. But the group remained positive, urging him to stay with the process and see where it might lead.

The dream group members began to ask questions about the pastel colors. What did they look like? Did they move and change—or did they stay the same? Did they just float in space, or were they part of a scene? With each question, the man shrugged and didn't have much to add. Then someone asked, "So how do you *feel* about pastel colors?"

That was the cue—the question that struck a chord. The man immediately replied, "I feel like they're weak. Washed out. Uncommitted. Pastel colors don't make me feel very good." The gentle probing continued. Is there any place in your life where you feel like that? Washed out? Uncommitted?

In short order it was revealed that the young man was studying to become a priest—he was a *pastoral* student. But that vocation wasn't his idea—it came from his family. It wasn't something to which he was deeply committed. Rather, it was something he felt was expected of him. His heart and soul weren't in it. He was uncommitted and felt, deep inside, like he was taking his life in the wrong direction to make other people happy. For him, *pastel* was a code word for "pastoral," and his feelings of weakness and unease about pastel colors formed a bridge that the dream was able—with the help of the group—to bring to consciousness, leading to a realization he was too embarrassed to consciously make for himself.

Philosophers might argue whether the original dream fragment of pastel colors intrinsically meant that the man felt weak and uncommitted about becoming a priest. But what is significant is that the combination of the dream—as fragmentary as it may have been—with the conscious process of group dream work created an opportunity for the man to reevaluate his life's path. This is not the same as an externally imposed analysis of the dreams supposed *a priori* meaning—whether in Biblical or Freudian terms. Pastel colors might have meant something totally different to another dreamer—for example, positive feelings about having a baby or a feeling of deep relaxation. But this type of dream work—precisely because it doesn't impose a fixed meaning on the contents of a dream—offers an opportunity for unique and deep personal discovery. The conclusions about his life that the young man reached were valid because, with the assistance of the group, they arose from the dreamer himself and resonated with his own sense of personal truth.

Why Do We Dream?

It is a common experience that a problem difficult at night is resolved in the morning after the committee of sleep has worked on it.

—John Steinbeck

There are many explanations of why we dream, and most fall into one of two broad categories—physiological reasons and psychological rationalizations. The physiological explanations center on how our bodies and brains function during the REM phase of sleep. Advocates of physiological explanations contend that we dream to exercise the synapses—the junctions that allow the transfer of messages from one neuron to another or from a neuron to another kind of cell.

They believe that dreaming takes over where the waking brain leaves off. When we're awake, our brains are busy transmitting and receiving messages, which traverse billions of cells to reach their destinations. Activation patterns are constantly shifting, and connections are constantly being made and unmade in our brains, forming the physical basis for our minds and cognitive processes. When we're dreaming, mental activity becomes less focused, looser, and is filled with imagery guided by the emotions of the dreamer.

Supporters of the physiological explanation of dreaming cite the fact that during the time of the greatest REM sleep, we experience the greatest number of dreams. Another observation that lends credence to this theory is that during REM sleep, EEG activity of the brain resembles the activity seen when we're awake but resting.

Psychological explanations of dreams focus on our thoughts and emotions, and posit that dreams help us to understand and negotiate the immediate concerns in our lives, such as unfinished business from the day or issues we are either incapable of handling or unwilling to deal with. Supporters of the psychological origin of dreams assert that dreams are not random; they are guided by the emotions of the dreamer and can teach us about our motivations, desires, and fears.

When we dream in response to a single, unambiguous emotion, it is often easy to identify the emotion involved and decipher the imagery and action in the dream. For example, survivors of traumas such as violent attacks or natural disasters often have dreams that depict the emotional response to the trauma, rather than the trauma itself. Their dreams recapitulate their feelings of terror or helplessness.

When dreams arise in response to several emotions or issues simultaneously, they become more challenging to decipher. Research reveals that intense dreams occur more frequently after trauma. This leads researchers to believe that the intensity of dream imagery is often a reliable measure of the emotional state of the dreamer.

Research conducted about dreams after traumatic or stressful events sheds additional light on this mysterious phenomenon. Someone who has just survived an earthquake may dream about the event a few times, and then may dream about being engulfed and drawn into the depths of the earth. In the weeks following the trauma, the dreams gradually connect the earthquake with other traumatic or stressful experiences the dreamer may have suffered in the past. The dreams then gradually return to their usual quality and duration.

Researchers hypothesize that these dreams act to connect recent traumatic experiences to past traumas in order to help us deal with the fresh trauma. By doing this, they alleviate some of the emotional disturbance associated with the trauma. When the traumatic material is connected with other parts of the memory system so that it no longer feels unique or extreme, the next time something similar occurs, the connections will already be present and the event will not feel quite so traumatic. This function of dreams may have been more important in earlier times, when people experienced trauma more frequently than those of us living in the developed world do today.

This hypothesis—that dreams are an adaptive mechanism that helps us cope with present and future traumas by weaving new material into the memory system in a way that reduces its emotional impact—is known as the contemporary theory of dreaming. There are many other, more complicated, explanations for dreams, including the prophetic nature of dreams described in the Bible, which is a belief shared by many cultures. Sigmund Freud, one of the fathers of modern psychology, believed dreams were symbolic of unresolved issues and conflicts buried deep within our minds and our memories. He deemed them "safety valves" for unconscious desires and called dreaming "the royal road to the unconscious."

DREAM ON

The physiological and psychological theories of dreaming are not necessarily in conflict. While some biologists, like DNA pioneer Francis Crick, have dismissed dreams as the result of "neurological garbage collection," it's important to remember that the human mind has a unique predisposition to create order from disparate sensory and cognitive information.

For example, we unconsciously link the separate frames of a motion picture into a perception of continuous movement. In a wide range of perceptual phenomena, we automatically and unconsciously "connect the dots" to construct patterns where only their outlines are actually provided. Many well-known

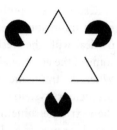

Kanizsa triangle

optical illusions such as the Kanizsa triangle shown here are based on this fact. In this illustration, our perceptual system creates the illusion of a triangle, even though none is actually present.

It's also one of the reasons why the testimonies of eyewitnesses to a crime are often contradictory—we tend to connect the dots to form patterns that resemble what we already expect. Different people, with different perceptions, biases, and points of view tend to build different narratives out of the same objective material.

One interesting perspective about the meaning of our dreams is the belief that every dream always contains elements that are uniquely personal—that is, specific to the individual dreamer—as well as other elements that are archetypal or transpersonal—that is, based on universal emotional and spiritual themes.

While Sigmund Freud tended to focus on the personal nature of dreams, reading in them a wealth of suppressed sexual drives and other types of wish fulfillment, his more spiritually focused contemporary Carl Jung looked more at the archetypes suggested by our dreams.

Archetypes are images, symbols, characters, and personalities that can be found in the literature, religions, and traditions of all cultures throughout history. In a sense, archetypes can be thought of as providing a fundamental, symbolically encoded vocabulary of the human experience.

For example, every culture has the archetype of the trickster. In Norse mythology, the trickster's name was Loki, and he was forever playing tricks on gods and humans alike—often with lethal consequences. In Native American lore, the trickster is sometimes called Coyote, associated with the spirit totem of that animal. In medieval German lore, the trickster was embodied by the irrepressible Till Eulenspiegel. We may know the trickster on a more personal level as the class clown—the nonconformist who acts out through humor or the creation of chaos, as opposed to the archetypical rebel who also may play tricks and facilitate dissent but does so with a more serious or melancholy disposition.

We often see archetypes reflected most clearly in organized systems of divination such as the tarot deck or the ancient Chinese oracle, the *I Ching*. Each of the tarot cards encodes a wealth of archetypal information in highly symbolic ways that parallel many aspects of dream experience. The *I Ching* derives from Taoist philosophy and bases its archetypes on the cycles of nature and the organization of human relationships. These and other ancient and traditional systems provide a way to touch deeply felt aspects of human experience while bypassing many of the ways in which the logical, waking mind attempts to impose a certain type of linear order.

Remembering our image of the kaleidoscope and the ways in which conscious dream work can often help us connect the content of our dreams with insights that are personally significant, it may be helpful to shift our point of view between the personal and transpersonal—between the perspective unique to the dreamer and the perspective of archetypal, transpersonal symbols.

EITHER/AND

Dreaming permits each and every one of us to be quietly and safely insane every night of our lives.

—Dr. William Dement, pioneering sleep researcher

We all know that many things in life present us with either/or decisions. Either I'm going to stay up late and finish this chapter *or* I'm going to get a good night's sleep and try to finish it tomorrow. Either I'm going to stick to my diet *or* I'm going to eat that beguiling hunk of chocolate fudge cake. Life constantly presents us with a stream of situations where choosing one thing eliminates a mutually exclusive choice. In fact, the origin of the word *decide* means "to cut off." Choose one option and you cut off all the others.

One of the most puzzling aspects of our dreams is that we often experience situations that, from the perspective of our waking minds, *should* work in this either/or fashion but which instead somehow take two or more paths—a phenomenon we can call either/and. In dreams, it's common to both have your cake and eat it too. During a dream, we experience no contradiction but, upon awakening, it can be difficult to put these experiences into language which is, by its nature, linear. We find ourselves saying things like, "I went up into the mountains to go hiking but, somehow, in a way I can't really explain, I was also at my office. I was talking to the president of the United States on the phone and watching the bald eagle eggs hatch. Then I was flying with the birds over the chasm even though I was still on the phone."

Language is a magnificent tool. It allows us to describe our thoughts and feelings to one another. It enables us to record information for posterity—histories, ideas, experiences, even recipes, blueprints, and other practical knowledge that our ancient ancestors struggled to attain and impart to future generations. But the price that we pay for this remarkable ability is that we have to funnel a network of connected thoughts and impressions into a linear sequence of words. We have created many ways to integrate flexibility into our narratives. Magazine articles and textbooks frequently use sidebars that sit outside the main flow of text. In language itself, we can make parenthetical comments or use imagistic language to suggest nonlinear connections. But when all is said and done, language is essentially linear, and our perception of choice is basically either/or.

This conflict between the essential nonlinearity of dreaming and the fundamental linearity of language may go a long way to explaining why so many people find it hard to remember their dreams. The attempt to shoehorn the dream narrative into the structures of language can be messy and frustrating. Some people may, unconsciously, prefer to dismiss their dream experiences rather than challenge their well-ordered, linearly structured waking realities.

Quantum Consciousness

At the beginning of the twentieth century, the way that scientists perceived the world changed in a fundamental way. As physicists began to explore the realm of the very small—at the level of individual atoms and the particles of which they're made—they discovered that our most basic notions of time and space no longer applied. At the so-called quantum scale, things could actually appear and disappear, be in many places at once, and even go backward and forward in time. These notions seem absurd to us because the collective action of countless quantum-scale particles adds up to the familiar behavior of the macroscopic world of human experience. But at the incredibly tiny level of atoms, the basic rules of reality are very different.

Interestingly, the either/and qualities of the dream state match very closely the behavior scientists observe at the quantum scale. The science of quantum mechanics—perhaps the most rigorously tested scientific theory in all human history—shows us that at the level of atoms and subatomic particles, the universe actually behaves more like either/and than either/or.

This is significant because some researchers working at the frontiers of biophysics (the intersection of biology, the study of living things, with physics, the study of the fundamental properties of the universe) have proposed that consciousness is actually a coherently organized quantum mechanical process. Physicists, including Sir Roger Penrose and the American anesthesiologist Dr. Stuart Hameroff, have proposed that our ordinary notions of reality are, in fact, built on top of a foundation of precisely organized quantum scale events.

Extreme Dreams

While many dreams are tough to remember, some are literally impossible to ignore.

Extreme dreams come in many forms, crashing into our sleeping minds with incredibly vivid imagery that can be at once terrifying, beautiful, or magically compelling. Some of these extreme dreams may arise from sleep deprivation, high fevers, brain injuries, or nervous system disorders, while others may actually be the subconscious mind's attempts to draw attention to issues, events, or actions of great personal importance. Elias Howe's nightmare about spears with holes at the end of them described at the beginning of this chapter is a perfect example of an important, positive message delivered in a form too shocking to ignore. We may fear or resist some types of extreme dreams, but they sometimes contain the seeds of great awakenings.

There are many types of exceptional dream states, some of which are so different from normal sleep and dreams they are considered to arise from different—and potentially pathological—stages of sleep. Some of us only experience these more extreme states of consciousness on rare occasions, if ever. Others, especially children, may experience them on a regular basis. Some, like nightmares, can be terrifying. Others, like hypnogogic or "twilight" states, lucid dreams, and so-called out-of-body experiences may at times be joyful and liberating.

Some types of extreme dream states include:

• **Nightmares.** Vivid and terrifying dreams that can powerfully capture our attention.

• **Twilight states.** Trance-like states often accompanied by beautiful sounds, images, and sensations such as flying or merging with objects—called hypnogogia if they occur while falling asleep and hypnopompia if they happen during the transition to waking.

• **Lucid dreams.** States in which the dreamer becomes aware of the dream, acquiring the ability to make conscious choices within the dream's unfolding narrative.

• **Out-of-body experiences**, sometimes called astral projection. Extraordinary states of awareness in which the domain of the dreamer's awareness becomes separated from the location of the physical body. Dreamers often have the experience of seeing their physical bodies left behind as they enter a different perceptual realm.

Because these states of consciousness can have such a huge impact on our awareness, a wide variety of psychological, spiritual, ritual, and magical explanations have arisen to explain them. While we may look askance at some of the more fantastic interpretations of these dreaming states, we should also be careful about simply reducing them to mere physiological anomalies or symptoms of illness and dysfunction.

In our earlier example of the young pastoral student who could only remember a vague dream of pastel colors, the perceived value of the dream emerged from the active process of working with it in the waking state, independent of whether the dream intrinsically contained the meanings typically discovered through dream work. Similarly, even though out-of-body experiences (or OOBEs for short) are often associated with abnormal neurological activity in the temporal lobes of the brain, the existence of these types of organic factors does not mean that the experience does not *also* have the ability to act as a powerful catalyst for psychological and spiritual exploration and transformation.

NIGHTMARES

It's probably safe to assume that everyone has, at some point in life, experienced the type of terrifying dream we call a nightmare. Nightmares may present themselves in the form of complex narratives featuring beasts or demons, or scenes of war, or other highly personal imagery. Most children experience nightmares at least occasionally—usually between the ages of about three and eight years of age. Sometimes, these nightmares correspond to traumatic events or stress factors, such as a divorce, family tensions, or the loss of a family member—even

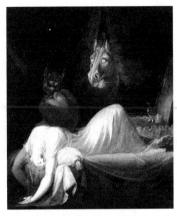

Nightmares can be terrifying.

a pet. Some nightmares are associated more directly with physical causes such as high fevers, injuries, or the use or rapid withdrawal of certain types of medications.

For most people, nightmares happen at most on an occasional basis. But sometimes, frequent or even recurring nightmares can become a significant problem. These problems may be physical, caused by the ongoing interruption of a healthy sleep cycle, or they may be psychological, creating emotional problems and anxieties that carry over into waking experience. In these cases, it's important to work with the nightmare situation, attempting first to identify and reduce possible physical causes such as illness or reaction to medications—and then, if necessary, to work with the emotional content of the nightmare experience.

In both children and adults, nightmares often emerge after experiences that challenge our emotional defenses. During the waking hours of the day, we have many distractions—work, school, friends, family—that may allow us to turn away from the memory of stressful or traumatic events. But at night, as our minds and bodies enter a state of repose, we may be less able to camouflage our raw, unresolved feelings with the white noise of other activities.

TWILIGHT STATES

Less common than nightmares—and usually far more pleasant—are the twilight states that some people experience during the transition from waking to sleeping (called hypnogogia, or hypnogogic experiences) and from sleeping to waking (called hypnopompia, or hypnopompic experiences). These transitional phases represent unusual, mixed states of consciousness in which many of the features of the waking mind are diminished or relaxed, similar to their status during regular phases of the sleep cycle, while others, including a vivid, heightened sense of perceptual awareness, continue to function and may even be enhanced. This unusual combination of mental states can give rise to feelings that subjectively seem enchanted or magical.

Different individuals experience these twilight states in distinctly different ways. Some may hear continuous streams of beautiful and complex music. In fact, this may be the origin of the "music of the spheres," an ancient concept that associates the geometry of the sun and planets with a universal, heavenly form of music experienced deep inside the body. While most philosophers through the ages have written about the music of the spheres as an abstract concept based on pure mathematics, some have insisted that they truly hear and deeply feel this music. It's quite possible that what they actually experienced was the translation of a mixed state of hypnogogic or hypnopompic consciousness into the subjective awareness of music.

Others who have experienced the twilight states report exceptionally vivid visual experiences—perhaps even being able to directly see objects at a microscopic level or observe scenes at a great distance, as though viewed through a telescope. Some people describe being able to look at an object and feel themselves projected directly into it. There are many reports that during twilight states people have the experience of effortlessly flowing up or down walls and even dematerializing and passing directly through them.

While many descriptions of these twilight states are benign or even pleasant, some twilight experiences have a darker aspect. Throughout history, there have been many reports of individuals experiencing "visitations" from grotesque, demonic, or seductive creatures. The most famous, perhaps, is the incubus, described as a male demon that preys upon sleeping women, taking advantage of their vulnerable state in order to have sexual relations with them.

This scenario has been richly embroidered over the centuries to include the notion that it is only through these nocturnal relations that the incubi can perpetuate their demonic species, draining vital energy from the women with whom they couple. The female version of the incubus is called the succubus—a demonic female who enters the sleeping world of a man in order to have sex with him. Most scholars believe that these demons are the result of widespread cultural attitudes of sexual repression and the demonization of sexual pleasure, which, during the uninhibited phases of sleep, may become manifest. Throughout history, reports of sexual relationships with succubi have been particularly common among celibate members of religious orders, where the rejection of sexuality and earthly pleasures are integral elements of the communal experience.

Because the hypnogogic and hypnopompic twilight states are more vivid, sensual, and difficult to repress than ordinary dreams, it is easier for these twilight experiences to become confused with waking reality.

LUCID DREAMS

The simplest, most direct definition of lucid dreaming comes from Stephen LeBerge, one of the leading researchers in the field. According to LeBerge, lucid dreaming is "dreaming while knowing that you are dreaming." In a sense, a lucid dream combines many of the familiar and fantastical elements of the conventional dream state with a level of conscious control we typically associate with waking states of consciousness. Lucid dreamers may use this awareness to work through personal challenges faced in the course of their waking lives or to explore experiences not available in the waking state, such as flying.

The first account of a lucid dream available to modern scholars is a letter from the fifth century written by Augustine of Hippo, one of the central figures in the development of Christianity.

A modern assessment of lucid dreaming that recognizes its scientific and therapeutic potential began in 1968 with the publication of Celia Elizabeth Green's book *Lucid Dreams* (Institute of Psychophysical Research, 1968). In it, Green argues that lucid dreams represent a distinctly different form of consciousness than ordinary dreaming and predicts that they are closely associated with REM sleep—an assertion that subsequent research has proven to be correct. She also associated lucid dreaming with another puzzling phenomenon called "false awakening" or "double dreaming." This is a situation in which the dreamer believes himself to have awakened but has, in fact, falsely awakened into another dream state.

In addition to providing a unique window into the relationships between the dreamer's subjective reality and the associated activities of the brain and nervous system, there may also be practical, therapeutic applications of lucid dreaming. For example, if an individual can learn to consciously step into the arena of the dream and assert a level of conscious control, then he or she may be able to transform a terrifying experience into one far more comprehensible and manageable. Used as an adjunctive psychotherapeutic tool, lucid dreaming can help a person who feels helpless or out of control in waking life to explore ways in which to shift their deeply held beliefs, attitudes, and behaviors. The protected space of the dream world can help reframe experiences more positively. Individuals suffering from recurring nightmares may also find a way to transform their tortured, helpless feelings by learning to take conscious control of their dreams. In this way, the lucid dream state may actually represent a wonderful intrapsychic laboratory.

OUT-OF-BODY EXPERIENCES

An out-of-body experience is a state of consciousness in which an individual feels a separation between conscious awareness and the location of the physical body. In some cases, the person having the experience is able to turn back and look at the physical body, typically finding it in its sleeping position in bed—an instance of a larger phenomenon called autoscopy.

Robert Monroe, one of the pioneers in the field of out-of-body experiences, has cataloged, described, and learned to control and induce these experiences. Monroe refers to the place where the physical body exists as local zero. In his many writings, he goes on to describe higher-order locales that exist at successively further removes from the physical body's location. According to Monroe, individuals can learn to induce the out-of-body state and consciously move between different planes of experience, each with its own characteristic geography and inhabitants.

As bizarre as this theory no doubt sounds, spiritual traditions and shamanic practices across cultures, including those of many Native American tribes, very closely match Monroe's descriptions. The consistency of these experiences across many cultures and many periods of time argues strongly that whatever the out-of-body experience really is, it represents a phenomenon nearly as universal, if somewhat less common, than ordinary dreaming. Carlos Castaneda, the controversial anthropologist whose books describe his purported initiation with a Mexican Yaqui shaman, Don Juan, details an elaborate system of conscious travel through alternate realms of reality in his book *The Art of Dreaming* (HarperCollins, 1993).

One of the consistent hallmarks of the out-of-body experience is a subjective sensation that what is experienced in this state is as real as the ordinary waking state. For someone experiencing an OOBE, there is, quite simply, no sense of being in a dream. For this reason if no other, the OOBE represents a singular and very remarkable state of awareness.

Neurobiologists have shown that the so-called out-of-body experience can be reliably associated with, and induced by, stimulation of a part of the brain called the angular gyrus, a region at the side of the head occurring at the junction between the temporal and parietal lobes of the brain. In medical studies, researchers often find lesions in this area that may, in at least some cases, be sufficient to trigger this stimulation during sleep. In a waking person, stimulation of the angular gyrus also may create a powerful sensation of being watched from behind by someone closely mimicking the OOB experiencer's movements.

Out-of-body experiences may happen spontaneously and usually occur during sleep but occasionally take place during waking. OOBEs frequently connect with lucid dreams, nightmares, or other vivid, non-ordinary states of consciousness. An OOBE may be launched from a lucid dream following the dreamer's awareness of their dreaming state, or it may land in a lucid dream in which the dreamer can evaluate the subjective sense of having taken a journey away from the body.

OOBEs are frequently, but not always, associated with a well-known REM sleep phenomenon called sleep paralysis. The body is routinely paralyzed during ordinary REM sleep to prevent the muscles from physically acting out the dreamer's actions—walking, running, talking, or more potentially dangerous activities such as cooking or driving. During the OOBE and especially during the transition to waking, an individual may be aware of his or her surroundings but unable to mobilize the body. In other words, people experiencing OOBEs may consciously experience the sleep paralysis that is normally submerged in a non-aware sleeping state.

Whether one chooses to understand the out-of-body experience as a genuine spiritual awakening, a palpable astral projection into other realms of existence, or merely as an internal neurobiological experience of a virtual reality arising from the atypical stimulation of certain regions of the brain, to those who experience OOBEs, they may be a source of profound joy and a deep, nearly universal sense of connection and belonging.

Troubled Sleep

Insomnia is a gross feeder. It will nourish itself on any kind of thinking, including thinking about not thinking.

—Clifton Fadiman

Troubled sleep is somewhat arbitrarily divided into two broad classes—sleep problems and sleep disorders. Although there is considerable overlap between them, sleep disorders are generally considered more serious than sleep problems.

Examples of sleep problems include occasional difficulty falling asleep, waking frequently during the night, waking too early, waking feeling tired or unrefreshed, occasional snoring and snorting, and nightmares (the last of which was covered in chapter 3). Bruxism, another problem that can occur during sleep, is the habitual, involuntary grinding or clenching of the teeth, often in response to feelings of anger, stress, fear, or frustration. Jet lag is a common sleep problem that affects travelers across time zones, resulting in temporary fatigue, insomnia, headache, and other symptoms.

Of the more than seventy identified sleep disorders, the most frequently occurring are insomnia, narcolepsy, obstructive sleep apnea, and restless legs syndrome. We'll consider each of these common sleep disorders in depth in this chapter, along with snoring and children's troubled sleep.

Insomnia

Insomnia comprises a range of sleep difficulties including difficulty falling and staying asleep, waking up too early in the morning and feeling unrefreshed by sleep, as well as daytime sleepiness. People who suffer from insomnia also may experience daytime consequences of sleep deprivation, including feeling tired, lacking the energy to perform their usual routines, difficulty concentrating, and mood disturbances such as irritability, anxiety, or depression.

Insomnia is the single most common sleep disorder and often occurs in response to stress or other health complaints. As many as 40 percent of adults report at least one bout of insomnia in any given year, and about 15 percent say their insomnia is chronic or severe. The prevalence of insomnia increases with age and it is more common in women.

Acute episodes of insomnia are most frequently attributable to emotional stress, physical discomfort stemming from illness or injury (such as back pain or muscle aches), or environmental disturbances (such as noise, light, or uncomfortable temperatures). Travel, especially across time zones, can produce jet lag and transient insomnia.

Chronic insomnia refers to experiencing these problems at least three nights per week for one month or longer. It's often difficult to tease out a single cause of chronic insomnia, and it is thought to arise from several factors such as medical, neurological, and psychological disorders acting in concert.

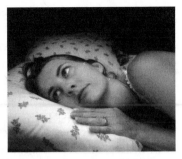
Insomnia is a common problem.

For example, some medical conditions such as gastroesophageal reflux (when stomach contents back up into the esophagus and cause heartburn) actually worsen when the sufferer lies down to sleep—the recumbent position mechanically increases the opportunity for reflux. The reflux sufferer may experience insomnia simply because of increased discomfort when reclining, or may be unable to fall asleep because of anxiety caused by anticipating increased discomfort or even anxiety about being unprepared to meet the challenges of the following day because of sleep deprivation.

Similarly, conditions such as benign prostatic hypertrophy (BPH)—a noncancerous growth of the prostate gland—prompt frequent awakenings and may produce insomnia, especially if the roused sleeper is unable to return to sleep. Anxiety about the condition and the anticipation of being awakened by the sudden need to urinate also may cause difficulties in falling asleep.

Other medical problems that may cause or contribute to chronic insomnia are conditions that may worsen at night, such as asthma and other breathing problems; hormonal shifts associated with pregnancy, perimenopause and menopause, chronic pain, and Alzheimer's disease and other dementias.

Nearly three-quarters of asthma patients report waking from sleep; some wake because their symptoms are aggravated at night, while others wake because their disease is poorly controlled. The drugs used to treat asthma also may contribute to sleep problems. Drugs used to treat asthma, including theophylline, β2-agonists, corticosteroids, and antihistamines, are known to alter sleep patterns.

Some asthma patients experience a change in the quality of their sleep, others note a change in the quantity of sleep— usually less—and still others find that anti-asthma drugs alter the continuity of their sleep, which results in broken sleep with frequent awakenings. The effects of anti-asthma drugs on sleep are patient dependent and may vary; for example, theophylline often causes disturbed sleep in adults with asthma (such as early morning awakening and daytime sleepiness), but it doesn't seem to disrupt sleep in asthmatic children.

Prescription Medications and Other Drugs

Prescription drugs, over-the-counter medications, and recreational drugs also may contribute to insomnia. Prescription medications with the potential to cause insomnia include antidepressants, beta blockers, decongestants, and steroids.

Antidepressants

At times prescribed for insomnia when it is thought that insomnia is linked to or stems from depression, antidepressants may themselves cause or worsen sleep disorders. Although some antidepressants such as tricyclic antidepressants (doxepin, amitriptyline, and trazodone) cause drowsiness, others often cause insomnia as a side effect. Monoamine oxidase inhibitors (MAOIs) such as phenelzine (Nardil) and tranylcypromine (Parnate) tend to cause sleep loss, as do antidepressants known as selective serotonin reuptake inhibitors (SSRIs), such as sertraline (Zoloft) and fluoxetine (Prozac).

BETA BLOCKERS

Prescribed to relieve stress on the heart, beta blockers slow the heartbeat, lessen the force with which the heart muscle contracts, and reduce blood vessel contractions in the heart, brain, and throughout the body. Beta blockers may cause nightmares and are thought to disrupt sleep by interacting with neurotransmitters such as serotonin. Beta blockers include acebutolol (Sectral), atenolol (Tenormin), metoprolol (Lopressor), nadolol (Corgard), pindolol (Visken), propranolol (Inderal), and timolol (Blocadren).

DECONGESTANTS

Commonly used to relieve congestion in the head and chest, as well as stuffy nose, runny nose, sinus problems, and allergy symptoms, decongestants are chemically related to adrenalin, which besides being a natural decongestant is also a stimulant. In addition to their use for cold, flu, and allergy symptoms, decongestants may be ingredients in over-the-counter diet pills. People who use decongestants or diet pills containing decongestants may experience periods of feeling nervous or jittery and may have trouble getting to sleep. Decongestants include phenylephrine (Neo-Synephrine) and pseudoephedrine (Sudafed).

STEROIDS

Steroids are prescribed to treat a variety of medical conditions ranging from hormonal imbalances and inflammatory conditions to managing the side effects of chemotherapy. Their use can create feelings of energy and heightened wakefulness. For this reason, patients prescribed steroids are often advised not to take them late in the day in order to prevent sleep problems. Steroids include prednisone and cortisol.

Alcohol, caffeine, nicotine, and recreational drugs, such as amphetamines, cocaine, and marijuana, all may contribute to insomnia.

When factors such as another chronic illness, pain, prescriptions, or nonprescription drugs are contributing causes of insomnia, researchers and clinicians call this sleep disorder secondary insomnia, or comorbid insomnia. While primary insomnia is not directly associated with any other health problem, it is most likely attributable to chronic stress, hyperarousal (heightened psychological and physiological tension that acts to produce reduced pain tolerance, anxiety, and exaggerated startle responses), or poor sleep hygiene. Sleep hygiene, which we'll consider later, describes the conditions and practices that promote continuous and effective sleep.

MIGHT INSOMNIA BE USEFUL?

Although most insomniacs are unhappy about their conditions, some people feel that they actually benefit from their insomnia—that it gives them a certain artistic or creative edge. They point to a long list of famous insomniacs including W.C. Fields, Charles Dickens, Marcel Proust, Marlene Dietrich, Marilyn Monroe, Vincent Van Gogh, Napoleon Bonaparte, Amy

Lowell, Alexandre Dumas, Judy Garland, Tallulah Bankhead, Franz Kafka, Theodore Roosevelt, Groucho Marx, Thomas Edison, Margaret Thatcher, and Mark Twain to support the contention that insomnia fuels drive, ambition, and creativity. (Supporters of this premise often fail to mention, however, that at least some of these celebrities famously battled their insomnia and may have lost, given that some of their deaths resulted from lethal combinations of drugs that were, at least in part, intended to help them sleep.)

At least one study supports the connection between creativity and insomnia. Researchers from the California State University at Fullerton studied sixty New Zealand children between the ages of ten and twelve, half of whom scored in the 90th percentile or better on a standard creativity test, while the other half fell short of that mark. The researchers' hypothesis was that there would be a higher incidence of sleep disturbance in highly creative children than in control children. The children completed questionnaires designed to identify and assess their sleeping habits. The results showed that there was a significant difference between the two groups, with the creative children reporting more sleep disturbance. The researchers tentatively concluded that these findings "suggest that creative ability may affect an individual's sleep patterns."

Narcolepsy

The National Institute of Neurological Disorders and Stroke (NINDS, part of the National Institutes of Health) defines narcolepsy as "a chronic neurological disorder caused by the brain's inability to regulate sleep-wake cycles normally. At various times throughout the day, people with narcolepsy experience fleeting urges to sleep. If the urge becomes overwhelming, patients fall asleep for periods lasting from a few seconds to several minutes. In rare cases, some people may remain asleep for an hour or longer."

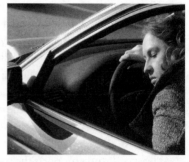
Narcolepsy can be hazardous.

Because narcoleptic sleep episodes can and do occur at any time, without warning, the condition can be disabling. While falling asleep while at work or at school may be inconvenient and distressing, falling asleep while driving or operating potentially hazardous machinery is life threatening.

Along with bouts of daytime sleepiness, people suffering from narcolepsy often experience cataplexy. Cataplexy may cause the sudden loss of voluntary muscle tone, vivid hallucinations while sleeping or immediately upon awakening, and brief but understandably terrifying attacks of complete paralysis while falling asleep or awakening. Because most people with narcolepsy have daytime drowsiness, periods of involuntary sleep, and frequent awakenings during nighttime sleep, narcolepsy is considered to be a disorder of the boundaries between sleep and wakefulness.

Although narcolepsy is not rare—about one in 2,000 Americans are affected—it is far less common than insomnia and other sleep disorders such as obstructive sleep apnea and restless legs syndrome. Most people who suffer from narcolepsy develop their first symptoms early in life, between the ages of ten and twenty-five, but the disorder can begin earlier and may develop at any stage in life.

As is the case for many diseases and neurological disorders, researchers believe that variants of certain genes and anatomical abnormalities in the brain predispose people to develop narcolepsy. Orexin, a blood peptide also known as hypocretin, is important in maintaining wakefulness and is absent in the brains of people who suffer from narcolepsy. Other factors may cause or contribute to the development of narcolepsy, including traumatic injuries to parts of the brain, tumors, infections, toxic exposures, stress, hormonal changes, and changes in sleep schedule. Recent research focuses on an immunological explanation of narcolepsy. NINDS-sponsored research has uncovered unusual immunological activity in dogs afflicted with narcolepsy.

The diagnosis of narcolepsy is often based on the patient's medical history and is confirmed using an overnight polysonogram and a multiple sleep latency test (MSLT). The MSLT is performed during the day to measure episodes of daytime sleep. The test subject takes four or five short naps during the course of a day. The MSLT measures the amount of time it takes for a person to fall asleep as well as heart and respiratory rates and nerve activity in muscles.

Although narcolepsy cannot be cured, its symptoms—daytime sleepiness, microsleeps, and cataplexy—can be managed using prescription drugs. Historically, physicians have prescribed stimulants such as amphetamines to prevent sleep attacks; however, these drugs can cause many undesirable side effects, including irritability and nervousness, shakiness, irregular heart rhythm, nighttime sleep disruption, and loss of appetite. There also is the potential for patients to develop tolerance with long-term use, leading to the need to increase the dose to maintain comparable levels of effectiveness.

A non-amphetamine drug—modafinil—overcomes some of the disadvantages of amphetamines and was approved for use by the Food and Drug Administration (FDA) in 1999. Modafinil doesn't have the problem with tolerance over long-term use. For many patients, tricyclic antidepressants and SSRIs help to control cataplexy.

Since medication improves but does not entirely eliminate daytime sleepiness, many people with narcolepsy also use other strategies such as scheduled daytime naps to prevent sleep attacks. They also try to improve the quality of their nighttime sleep (see chapter 6 for more on sleep hygiene) and take special safety precautions, especially when driving or operating machinery. The NINDS reports that while people with untreated narcolepsy are involved in automobile accidents about ten times more often than the general population, the rates of accidents among persons with narcolepsy who are on an effective treatment regimen are comparable to the general population.

Obstructive Sleep Apnea

If you snore loudly and often, wake up gasping for breath, and suffer from daytime sleepiness, then you may have sleep apnea. Sleep apnea is a condition in which breathing becomes very shallow or stops completely for short periods during sleep. Each pause lasts about ten to twenty seconds or longer, and pauses can occur twenty times or more an hour. Sleep apnea can increase the risk of developing high blood pressure, heart attack, or stroke. Untreated, sleep apnea can increase the risk of diabetes and daytime sleepiness. The resulting difficulty in concentration from daytime sleepiness can increase the risk for automobile and work-related accidents.

Recent research also reveals that sleep apnea is strongly associated with depression. A population-based study funded by the NIH found that the more severe the sleep apnea, the greater the risk for depression. It also showed that treating sleep apnea helped to prevent and relieve depression. The researchers speculated that the fragmented sleep and intermittent lack of oxygen to the brain may either cause or contribute to the development of depression.

Apnea literally means "to stop breathing," and there are two types of sleep apnea—central and obstructive. Central sleep apnea, in which the signals to the muscles involved in breathing do not function properly, is much less common than obstructive sleep apnea (OSA). In central sleep apnea, breathing may also be disrupted during wakefulness because the nerves do not always carry the correct signals from the brain to the muscles.

In persons with obstructive sleep apnea, during sleep there is insufficient airflow into the lungs through the mouth and nose, and the amount of oxygen in the blood may drop because the airway is transiently blocked.

According to the National Heart, Lung, and Blood Institute, more than twelve million Americans have obstructive sleep apnea, and one in twenty-five men over age forty and one in fifty women over age forty have debilitating sleep apnea that causes them to be very sleepy during the day. The condition is more common in men, African Americans, Hispanics, and Pacific Islanders. An estimated eighteen million Americans have sleep apnea, and while sleep apnea has been diagnosed more frequently in recent years, researchers contend that as many as 90 percent of patients remain undiagnosed and untreated.

Obesity, particularly upper body obesity, is a risk factor for OSA and is related to its severity. Many people with sleep apnea have a body mass index (BMI) greater than thirty. (BMI is a key index for relating a person's body weight to their height that offers a general indication if weight falls within a healthy range; BMI over twenty-five is considered overweight and over thirty is considered obese.)

In general, men whose neck circumference is seventeen inches or greater and women with a neck circumference of sixteen inches or greater are at higher risk for sleep apnea. Large neck girth in both men and women who snore is highly predictive of sleep apnea because persons with large neck girth store more fat around their necks, which may compromise their airways. A smaller airway can make breathing difficult or stop it altogether. In addition, fat stored in the neck and throughout the body can produce substances that cause inflammation, and inflammation in the neck may be a risk factor for sleep apnea. Weight loss usually resolves or significantly improves sleep apnea by decreasing neck size and reducing inflammation.

Anatomic risk factors for obstructive sleep apnea run in families—the volume of upper-airway soft tissue structures, including the lateral pharyngeal walls and tongue, is greater in individuals with OSA than in healthy control subjects. Family history of OSA explains about 30 percent of the variability of OSA in the general population and an individual with a first-degree relative with OSA has a 50 to 75 percent higher risk of having the condition than an individual with no known affected relatives. Researchers postulate the existence of a syndrome involving obesity, high blood pressure, and diabetes, in which OSA exacerbates the other traits, generating a vicious cycle.

A large, ten-year prospective controlled study of untreated men with severe obstructive sleep apnea followed 264 healthy men, 377 men who simply snored, 403 with untreated mild to moderate OSA, 235 with severe OSA, and 372 with treated severe OSA. Treated subjects with OSA had fatal and non-fatal cardiovascular event rates (heart attack, hypertension, and stroke) that were closer to those seen in healthy subjects than the subjects with severe OSA that went untreated. Subjects with untreated severe OSA had two to three times the risk of fatal and non-fatal cardiovascular events compared with healthy subjects. The investigators concluded that there is a relationship between the severity of OSA and cardiovascular risk, but effective treatment with continuous positive airway pressure (CPAP) seems to cut this risk and significantly reduce cardiovascular illness associated with OSA.

Sleep apnea is diagnosed based on a complete medical history, physical examination, and sometimes a sleep study, which involves a polysonogram recording which may be performed in the hospital, at an outpatient clinic, or at home. The sleep study records brain activity, eye movement, muscle activity, breathing and heart rates, how air moves in and out of the lungs during sleep, and the percentage of oxygen in the subject's blood during an entire night's sleep.

There are several treatment options for OSA. Mild OSA may be relieved by weight loss or by sleeping on one side, rather than on the back, because sleeping on the side may help the throat to remain open during sleep. Some OSA sufferers may benefit from special devices such as oral appliances or custom-fitted mouthpieces. Others gain relief from surgery such as procedures that remove the tonsils and adenoids if they are blocking the airway or uvuloplatopharyngoplasty (removal of tonsils, uvula [the tissue that hangs from the back of the roof of the mouth], and part of the soft palate) to correct the obstruction.

CPAP is the most common treatment for OSA. This treatment involves wearing a mask over the nose during sleep, which is connected to a machine that blows air into the throat at a pressure level calibrated for the individual CPAP user. The increased airway pressure keeps the throat open during sleep. People with sleep apnea should never take sedatives or sleeping pills, which can prevent them from awakening enough to breathe.

Restless Legs Syndrome

Restless legs syndrome (RLS) is a disorder that produces disagreeable creeping, crawling, prickling, burning, or tingling sensations in the calves, thighs, and feet and an overwhelming urge to move them to relieve these unpleasant sensations. The unpleasant sensations usually begin while people are inactive—sitting or lying down for prolonged periods of time—and typically symptoms worsen at night. Moving the legs eases the feelings, but only for a while.

There is a known circadian rhythm to RLS. Sleep studies reveal that people with RLS often obtain the most beneficial and restorative sleep later in the twenty-four-hour cycle—such as from 2 a.m. to approximately 10 a.m.

RLS is one of the most common sleep disorders, especially among older adults. About 12 million Americans suffer from

RLS, enduring constant leg movement during the day and insomnia at night. Although symptoms may develop at any age and RLS may be associated with other health conditions such as anemia, pregnancy, or diabetes, the most severe cases occur in persons over age sixty-five.

Many RLS patients also suffer from a related disorder known as periodic limb movement disorder (or PLMD), which causes repetitive jerking movements of the limbs, especially the legs. People with PLMD experience jerking movements as often as every twenty to forty seconds, which make it difficult to fall asleep and, naturally, wake them from sleep.

The diagnosis of RLS is generally made on the basis of a physical examination and medical history. Although there's no diagnostic test specifically for the diagnosis of RLS, physicians often check blood ferritin (iron) levels and may, if needed, suggest supplementing the diet with iron, vitamin B12, or folate. Because RLS and PLMD symptoms are relieved by drugs (such as pramipexole [Mirapex], pergolide [Permax], ropinirole [Requip], and a combination of carbidopa and levodopa [Sinemet]) that affect the neurotransmitter dopamine, researchers think that the condition may result from an imbalance of dopamine, which sends messages to control muscle movement. Other drug treatment includes the use of narcotics, muscle relaxants, and sleep medications, as well as treatment with gabapentin (Neurontin), a drug that is often prescribed to treat epilepsy.

People with mild-to-moderate RLS frequently find relief in simple medical self-care measures. Along with avoiding caffeine, alcohol, tobacco, and other substances that have the potential to disrupt sleep and taking over-the-counter pain relievers such as ibuprofen (Advil, Motrin) or naproxin sodium

(Aleve) when symptoms begin, many RLS sufferers find they can calm symptoms using the following treatments:

HEAT

Hot baths and alternating heat and cold often help to relieve unpleasant sensations. Heat can relax the muscles, improve blood flow and help to reduce overall stress and tension.

COUNTERSTIMULI

Massage and other activities that provide counterstimuli such as such as applying vibration or acupressure or stretching or jiggling the affected limbs may provide temporary relief of symptoms.

RELAXATION TECHNIQUES

Relaxation techniques such as meditation and yoga have been found to help many RLS sufferers cope with the disorder.

EXERCISE

Exercise improves circulation and muscle tone and can help to manage stress.

TRANSCUTANEOUS ELECTRIC NERVE STIMULATION

Transcutaneous electric nerve stimulation (TENS) helps to reduce nighttime leg movements by applying electrical stimulation to an area of the feet or legs. The therapy is performed for fifteen to thirty minutes before bedtime.

Snoring

There ain't no way to find out why a snorer can't hear himself snore.
—Mark Twain

Snoring occurs when air flows past relaxed tissues in your throat, causing the tissues to vibrate as you breathe and generating husky growls and rasping sounds. The sounds of snoring are quite distinctive, which is why it's often called "sawing logs." About 40 percent of adults snore, and snoring is more common in men than women. For most, it's just a minor problem, but for some people, loud, unrelenting snoring can be a sign of a serious medical condition. For others, noisy snoring followed by seconds in which breathing stops is the hallmark of obstructive sleep apnea.

Snoring keeps other people awake even when it doesn't compromise the quality of sleep of the snoring person, and it often hampers their relationships. A 2005 National Sleep Foundation survey found that 30 percent of survey respondents with a snoring or easily awakened partner said they felt snoring had harmed their relationships. Partners of people who snore may find that earplugs are the most important investment they can make to ensure uninterrupted sleep.

Most snoring is attributable to the anatomy of the mouth and throat. People who snore are more likely to have low, thick, soft palates or enlarged tonsils or tissues in the back of their throats that narrow or constrict their airways. If the uvula is longer than usual, airflow may be obstructed and vibration increased. The more vibrations that occur, the more likely you'll be considered a snorer. People who are overweight or obese are more likely to have narrowed airways.

In other instances, snoring may be due to nasal congestion or obstruction from a cold, flu, allergy, or other respiratory condition, or an anatomical problem such as a deviated nasal septum. The nasal septum is a thin structure that separates the two sides of the nose. When it is sufficiently displaced to one side ("deviated" from the symmetrical middle), the flow of air and mucus are impeded.

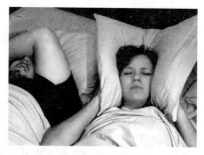

A partner's snoring can be disruptive to getting a good night's sleep.

Alcohol consumption as well as some prescription drugs such as sedatives also may be implicated in snoring. Alcohol relaxes the muscles in the throat, which in turn increases the likelihood of snoring.

Snoring can often be diminished by weight loss, avoidance of alcohol in the evening, and sometimes by something as simple as changing your sleeping position—people who sleep on their backs are advised to try side sleeping to prevent snoring. Nasal strips that stick to the outside of the nose help many snorers to increase the size of their nasal passages while they sleep, which in turn eases breathing.

When these measures fail, oral appliances—form-fitting dental mouthpieces that help advance the position of the tongue and soft palate to keep the air passage open—can help to prevent snoring. Surgical interventions to treat snoring include uvulopalatopharyngoplasty, a procedure intended to tighten up flabby tissues and enlarge the upper air passages; laser-assisted uvulopalatoplasty, in which a laser is used to shorten the soft palate and remove the uvula; and radio frequency tissue ablation (somnoplasty), in which low-intensity radio frequency signals are used to remove part of the soft palate.

Children Have Sleep Problems, Too

Average daily sleep requirements decrease with age from a high at birth of 16.5 hours per day to twelve hours at age three, ten hours at age nine and nine hours per day for teens. Still, many children and teens suffer from sleep problems that prevent them from getting the amount of sleep they need for healthy growth as well as optimal performance in school, sports, and life in general.

The most common sleep problem among children from infancy through the school-age years involves making the wake-to-sleep transition independently—without parents calming them. Many parents use a variety of soothing-to-sleep behaviors, such as nursing, bottle feeding, rocking, holding, pacifiers, and car rides, which may inadvertently lead to sleep problems. As a result of being soothed to sleep, some infants don't learn how to self-soothe and require specific environmental cues to fall asleep. As they learn to fall asleep without the comfort of rocking or a bottle, parents also learn to gradually wean children from the expectation of intervention.

Infants also may learn to expect feedings during the night and will wake to this cue, which can become a self-perpetuating cycle. If this learned hunger is permitted to persist beyond infancy, then it can cause ongoing sleep disturbances. Many parents find that spacing feedings at longer intervals and tapering amounts at each feeding help babies learn to feel hunger less frequently and awaken less frequently during the night.

Toddlers often try to stall at bedtime, and can use a variety of creative tactics to avoid going to sleep. When parents fail to calibrate their children's expectations about bedtimes and bedtime rituals and give in to toddlers' every request, both the child and parent may suffer sleep loss. Clear expectations and limit setting can help toddlers to make the transition to sleep more easily. In fact, they benefit from many of the same routines and rituals associated with good sleep hygiene for adults (see chapter 6 for more information on sleep hygiene).

Other common problems that children may face at bedtime include fears or feeling scared at night. Many young children are afraid of the dark, of being alone, or even of routine noises in the house. Night lights, sleeping with a transitional object such as a beloved stuffed animal or blanket, and reassurance from parents are often sufficient to quell these fears. Life changes, such as starting a new school, moving, divorce, illness, or death in the family, also may precipitate sleep problems.

Similarly, even young children are as likely to suffer from worry and stress as adults. The pressures of school, exams, athletic competitions, and relationships can cause anxiety that interferes with sleep. Teenagers face additional pressures and may lose sleep over midterms, finals, and the stressful process of completing college applications.

Less often, children suffer from parasomnias—night terrors or nightmares brought on by sleep deprivation, irregular sleep-wake cycles, anxiety, frightening or traumatizing experiences, or medical illnesses. Bed-wetting, sleep apnea, narcolepsy, asthma, depression, and restless legs syndrome also occur in children and adolescents and can seriously disrupt sleep.

Older children and adolescents tend to be sleep deprived for many of the same reasons adults do—they are overscheduled. Children and teens may sacrifice sleep to complete homework, to participate in extracurricular activities, or to stay up late to watch television, play video games, or exchange instant messages with friends online. Sleep deprivation can have a cumulative effect, and sleep deprived students may miss school or arrive late, fall asleep in class, or suffer from irritability, diminished concentration, and fatigue. Sleep-deprived children also may suffer more illnesses than their well-rested peers.

Parents are often unaware that their children are suffering from sleep deprivation. In general, signs that children need more sleep than they are getting include:

- Needing to be awakened in the morning for school or day care

- Sleeping two or more hours on weekends and vacations than they normally do on school days

- Falling asleep at school or soon after arriving home

- Behaviors and moods that differ dramatically on days when they get more sleep

Between 5 and 10 percent of adolescents suffer from delayed sleep phase syndrome (DSPS), which is a circadian rhythm disorder. In DSPS, habitual sleep-wake times are delayed by two or more hours beyond the desired bedtime. Affected teens report that they simply can't fall asleep until two or three in the morning no matter how hard they try. If, however, they go to sleep at those early morning hours, then they fall asleep immediately. Once asleep, adolescents with DSPS have normal sleep quality. DSPS usually becomes a problem when affected teens are chronically late or absent from school.

Treatment for DSPS requires motivated and disciplined teens that are willing to adhere to a consistent sleep schedule seven nights a week. Using a technique known as phase advancement, they advance their bedtime fifteen minutes every few nights or as soon as they can easily fall asleep at the earlier time. Once the desired bedtime is attained, the teenager must keep strictly to the new sleep schedule, because even a single night off the schedule can cause a return to the delayed sleep phase pattern. Some teens with DSPS also benefit from melatonin to help advance their circadian clocks.

Help Children Learn to Manage Stress

A ruffled mind makes a restless pillow.

—Charlotte Brontë

Teaching children to effectively manage stress and become resilient early in life will help to immunize them against the harmful consequences of stress throughout their lives. Resilience does not entirely eliminate or reduce stress; it simply equips the child to engage differently with stressors. Children who learn to overcome obstacles and withstand pressures will be better able to make healthy choices throughout their lives.

Along with leading by example—modeling positive ways to deal with stress—researchers and mental health professionals feel there are many ways for parents to help build children's resilience. The efforts can begin at birth. Recent research reveals that breast-fed children are better able to cope with stress than their bottle-fed peers. Investigators tracked the health of nearly nine thousand boys and girls born in the United Kingdom in 1970. In 1980, when the children were ten years old, the investigators assessed their ability to cope with stress by looking at how they were affected by family problems. They found that children who were bottle-fed were more than four times as stressed by such events than those who were breast-fed.

Although the mechanism whereby breastfeeding confers stress resistance is not completely understood, it may be that the close bond forged between mother and child during breastfeeding fosters a sense of security that enables children to better manage stress in later life. In addition, the hormones present in breast milk may not only reduce stress in the nursing infant but also nourish the parts of the brain involved in managing stress. Research about how to raise stress-resistant children shows that babies who get plenty of attention in infancy develop the security and self-confidence necessary to overcome adversity later. Children develop resilience when offered opportunities in which they struggle to achieve success and feel the satisfaction of accomplishment. Parents, teachers, and other adults in their lives can help children identify the activities and pastimes that give them personal pleasure and those that help them to feel calm and relaxed. Like adults, children benefit from social connectedness, and having supportive family members and a network of friends provides a buffer against stress.

Children can be taught to reduce their stress and anxiety and to transform fear of change into anticipation. Identifying sources of stress—exams, team tryouts, conflicts with friends—and talking with children about how to resolve problems also helps build resilience.

Today's children are often overscheduled—juggling home and work with after-school sports, music lessons, and playdates. It is just as important for children as it is for adults to have quiet time. Focusing on just one or two extracurricular activities may free up some much needed leisure time. Allowing children some measure of control over their time—to choose how they spend their leisure time—also helps to instill the confidence and mastery that will help them to manage stress.

Other Common Sleep Disorders

Circadian Rhythm Disorders

These disorders relate to the timing of sleep within the twenty-four-hour day. Some of these disorders are related to the timing of sleep that the sleeper can control to some extent, such as shift work or time zone changes. Other circadian rhythm disorders have neurological origins. Examples of these are irregular sleep-wake pattern and advanced sleep phase syndrome, in which sufferers fall asleep well ahead of conventional or desired bedtimes and then wake too early.

Hypersomnia

Disorder characterized by much more sleepiness than is usual, including longer duration of nighttime sleep, unplanned daytime sleep, and an inability to remain awake or alert.

Parasomnias

From *para,* meaning "around" and *somnia*, meaning "sleep," these are sleep disorders in which unusual, and at times dangerous, events interfere with sleep. Such events include night terrors, sleep talking, sleepwalking, nightmares, bed-wetting, sleep apnea, or nighttime seizures.

NIGHT TERRORS

Night terrors involve abruptly waking from sleep in a panicked and frightened state. They occur during deep sleep—stages 3 and 4—and often occur in response to emotional stress. They are more than simply extreme versions of nightmares—nightmares usually occur during REM sleep, while night terrors generally happen in the first half of the night. Most people, especially children, are unable to recall the details of the night terror; they simply wake frightened and confused, often in a sweat, with a rapid heart rate. Children ages three to five and preadolescent boys are the most frequent sufferers, and although they are difficult to console, given comfort and reassurance most children who experience night terrors outgrow them by early adolescence. When adults suffer night terrors, they are often attributable to unusual stress or alcohol or drug use.

SLEEPWALKING

Also known as somnambulism, sleepwalking is a type of parasomnia. In addition to walking while in a deep stage of sleep, it involves seemingly purposeful movements, such as dressing. Interestingly, when sleepwalkers are given sedatives before sleep, the drugs seem to intensify their nocturnal activities. It is important to take precautionary measures to prevent sleepwalkers from losing balance, tripping, or suffering other accidents and injuries. There is an enduring urban legend that says that it is dangerous or harmful to wake a sleepwalker. This is entirely untrue. Although sleepwalkers may appear groggy or confused when awakened during an episode, there is no harm in waking them, and doing so may help them to avoid unintentional injuries.

The Risks and Consequences of Sleep Deprivation

Sure, sleep deprivation can leave you feeling grumpy, listless, and unable to focus, but did you know that lack of sleep disrupts every physiological function in the body and that it could seriously harm your health?

Under strict experimental conditions, even short-term sleep deprivation produces a variety of adverse physiological effects, including high blood pressure, activation of the sympathetic nervous system, impairment of blood sugar control, and increased inflammation. A variety of epidemiologic (population) studies have also suggested an association between sleep duration and long-term health.

Chronic sleep deprivation has been implicated in the development of a number of illnesses and conditions, including high blood pressure and heart disease, obesity, diabetes, immune system problems, as well as poor performance in school, in the workplace, and during sports. Chronic sleep loss may also contribute to acceleration of the aging process.

Sleep serves as an indicator of physical and mental health and quality of life. Insufficient sleep is associated with poor decision-making, impaired judgment, and poor coordination, as well as increased risk-taking and delayed reaction time. All of these problems translate into serious safety risks such as impaired driving, car accidents, and other kinds of errors. Sleep deprivation can trigger or exacerbate anxiety, depression, and other emotional problems, and it can heighten the symptoms of disorders involving concentration and impulse control such as attention deficit hyperactivity disorder (ADHD).

The health hazards of sleep deprivation travel in both directions. Insufficient or poor sleep can have an adverse affect on health, and physical and mental health problems may exert a negative impact on the quality and duration of sleep. Complicating matters further, many prescription and over-the-counter medications used to treat physical and mental health problems associated with poor sleep may also cause insomnia or daytime sleepiness.

Heart Health

Lack of sleep, whether short-term sleep loss or chronic deprivation, can have a serious impact on cardiovascular health. Both blood pressure and heart rate increase following sleep-deprived nights.

Sleeping less than five or six hours per night has been linked to increased risk for high blood pressure. One study of subjects between the ages of thirty-two and fifty-nine found that sleeping less than five hours per night was associated with more than double the risk for high blood pressure. Other research has confirmed that men who sleep five hours or less a night suffer twice as many heart attacks as men who sleep eight hours or longer.

Sleep deprivation also increases the risk of heart disease in women. Women who sleep less than five hours a night have a 30 percent higher risk of developing coronary heart disease than those who sleep eight hours or longer. Although studies have also found that oversleeping is associated with a greater risk of heart disease, many researchers speculate that oversleeping is actually an indicator of other illnesses that increase risk for heart disease—such as such as sleep apnea—rather than a risk factor.

A sleep deficit can place the body on high alert, increasing the production of cortisol, a hormone produced principally in response to physical or psychological stress. Higher cortisol levels drive up blood pressure, a major risk factor for heart attacks and strokes. Moreover, people who are sleep-deprived have elevated concentrations of cholesterol, cytokines (proteins produced by white blood cells that act as chemical messengers between cells that appear in the blood in certain acute inflammatory conditions), and increased levels of C-reactive protein, an important marker for inflammation that plays a role in the initiation and progression of cardiovascular disease.

Inflammation can damage the inner walls of the arteries, leading to possible stroke or heart disease. Sleep influences the functioning of the lining of blood vessels. Blood pressure rises in the early morning hours, which may in part explain why people are most likely to suffer heart attacks and strokes during early morning hours.

A recent study found that even relatively healthy people

who suffer from sleep disruptions appear to have an increased chance of developing blood clots, known as thrombi, because disrupted sleep increases levels of prothrombotic factors, which are known to predict the risk of coronary artery disease.

In addition to increasing the risk of cardiovascular disease, a prolonged, heightened state of inflammation has also emerged as a significant risk factor for cancer and diabetes.

Cancer

When researchers discovered that shift workers who work through the night were unusually prone to breast and colon cancer, they identified one possible explanation: exposure to light at night reduces levels of the hormone melatonin, which the brain produces during sleep. Melatonin—an antioxidant that helps to counter the damage caused by free-radical compounds, including cancer-causing mutations—is also thought to protect against cancer by affecting levels of other hormones, such as estrogen.

Melatonin can prevent tumor cells from growing and slows the production of estrogen by the ovaries. In many cases of ovarian and breast cancer, estrogen stimulates the cancerous cells to continue dividing. Researchers hypothesize that people who are up late at night or get up frequently in the night on average produce less melatonin, which in turn means that more cancer-activating estrogen is circulating throughout their bodies.

Another by-product of sleep deprivation is a shifted cortisol rhythm. Cortisol usually peaks at dawn and declines throughout the day. Since cortisol helps to regulate immune system activity, including the activity of a group of immune cells called natural-killer cells (NK cells) that help to combat cancer, people whose cortisol cycle is disrupted by troubled sleep may be more likely to develop cancer.

Diabetes

Research reveals that chronically sleep-deprived people tend to develop problems regulating their blood sugar, which may increase their risk for diabetes. Studies also have demonstrated that sleep deprivation in healthy men results in disturbances of glucose metabolism.

Even healthy young adults who regularly get by on just five hours of sleep a night have to secrete 30 percent more insulin to regulate their blood glucose levels than their peers who sleep eight hours or longer. Chronic sleep deprivation is associated with impaired carbohydrate tolerance. This is at least in part because lack of sleep increases cortisol levels, which inhibit the body's ability to metabolize glucose. This in turn overworks the pancreas, leading to diabetes.

Many studies have confirmed a clear and direct relationship between sleep duration and insulin sensitivity—the capacity to respond to insulin-stimulated glucose uptake following consumption of carbohydrates. Short sleepers have lower insulin sensitivity, and longer sleepers have higher insulin sensitivity. One study found that men who slept four hours per night for six consecutive nights lose 30 percent of their ability to respond to insulin. Another found that just one week of sleep deprivation brought healthy volunteer subjects to a pre-diabetic state.

Immune System Functions

Sleep has powerful effects on immune function. Sleep deprivation has been shown to alter immune responses and to increase circulating blood levels of inflammatory markers such as interleukin IL-6, tumor necrosis factor (TNF) [alpha], and C-reactive protein, with measurable and significant elevations after only one night of sleep loss. Sleep deprivation is also correlated with a significant reduction in cellular immunity and can cause reductions in NK cells, T-cells and monocyte function.

Sleep loss has been shown to induce a functional alteration of the proinflammatory cytokine response. Even a modest amount of sleep loss—four hours—also alters molecular processes that drive cellular immune activation and induce inflammatory cytokines. The good news is that once sleep is recovered, the immune system seems to easily rebound. It's reasonable to suggest that improving sleep could potentially reduce inflammation and, by doing so, reduce the risk for inflammatory diseases.

Sleep also plays an important role in supporting adaptive cellular immune responses, which suggests that improving sleep could potentially be an important additional treatment for certain immunological disorders and enhance the benefits of immunization. In fact, there is recent evidence that sleep deprivation decreases the antibody response to the influenza vaccine. Men who slept just four hours per night for four consecutive nights after receiving a flu shot produced just half the antibodies as the control group that received eight or more hours per night.

Could Sleep Loss = Weight Gain?

Recent research reveals that sleep duration is related to weight gain. People who sleep the least appear to be the most likely to gain weight and to become overweight and obese, possibly because their sleep debts make them less able to control hunger and recognize satiety.

Even mild sleep deprivation quickly disrupts normal levels of serotonin, as well as leptin and ghrelin, the hormones that regulate appetite and satiety. Reduced levels of serotonin, which is associated with feeling pleasure, may prompt some people to compensate for sleep deprivation with food, especially carbohydrates, to provide a quick sugar rush. Ghrelin stimulates feelings of hunger—it is an appetite-stimulating hormone released mostly by the stomach. Leptin, considered a satiety or fullness hormone, is released by the fat cells and tells the brain about the current state of energy balance of the body. When leptin levels are high, the brain receives the message that the body has enough food, and you feel full, while low leptin levels increase appetite.

Sleep deprivation leads to decreased levels of the satiety hormone leptin, increased levels of the hunger hormone ghrelin, and impaired glucose tolerance. Volunteers subjected to partial sleep deprivation reported that their appetites increased, and researchers observed a high level of correlation between the subjects' assessments of their appetites and an increase in their ghrelin to leptin ratios.

Interestingly, the subjects' desire for high carbohydrate and calorie-rich foods skyrocketed while their appetite for protein-rich foods was essentially unaffected. One possible explanation for the increased consumption of carbohydrates is to supply the sleep-deprived brain with glucose, which it uses as fuel.

After sleeping just four hours, the ratio of ghrelin to leptin increased by 71 percent, compared to sleeping ten hours. As the subjects' appetites increased, their food choices changed. After two nights of sharply limited sleep the volunteers increased their consumption of foods such as candy, cookies, and cake, while their consumption of fruit, vegetables, and dairy products did not increase. These findings have prompted researchers to conclude that the neuroendocrine regulation of appetite and food intake appears to be influenced by sleep duration, and that sleep restriction may favor the development of obesity.

In fact, sleep deprivation might be one of the factors fueling the obesity epidemic in the United States. According to the North American Association for the Study of Obesity, more than two-thirds of Americans are overweight or obese, and while we know that obesity is largely due to overeating and too little physical activity, researchers question why we are eating so much.

Some researchers wonder if there is a link between the fact that so many of us are both sleep deprived and unable to tame our appetites for high carbohydrate, calorie-dense foods. The media and food manufacturers also have taken notice of Americans' changing sleep patterns, tempting night owls with television advertisements for fast food and extending the hours of drive-through windows so we can load up on fat, sugar, and other empty calories for midnight snacks. And late-night snacking can throw off our sleep-wake rhythms by providing ill-timed spikes of blood sugar and bursts of energy just when we should be sleeping.

Learning and Memory

It's easy to understand how sleep deprivation can seriously compromise your ability to learn. Sleepy people have trouble concentrating, their minds wander, and their response times slow. Lack of sleep reduces the ability to pay attention and slows the ability to think and react quickly, while increasing the likelihood of making mistakes. When we perform tasks after a few nights of sleeplessness, slower response times, fatigability (the deterioration of performance over time), impaired thinking, reduced learning, and short-term recall can be expected.

As we discussed briefly in chapter 1, memory—the retention of material that has been learned—is necessary in order for learning to occur. Memory involves the creation, use, and maintenance of strong networks of brain cells. Researchers report that areas of the brain activated during daytime learning were reactivated during sleep. Apparently, sleep is the brain's way of managing the connections, boosting some while reducing others. With reduced sleep, the brain doesn't have time to properly restore neural connections.

Pulling even a single all-nighter can triple reaction time and vastly increase lapses of attention. Researchers at the University of Pennsylvania studied subjects who had slept four, six, or eight hours per night for two weeks. Using a psychomotor vigilance task (which measures behavioral alertness through reaction times to a sustained attention task), the researchers assessed the subjects' speed of reaction to a computer screen counting up in milliseconds from zero to one second. Their first assignment was to recognize that the count had begun, then to stop it as quickly as possible by hitting a key.

The sleep-deprived subjects not only were somewhat slower than their well-rested peers, but they also had far more microsleeps—brief involuntary lapses—letting an entire second pass without responding. There also was a direct relationship between the duration of sleep and lapses—subjects with just four hours a night had more lapses than those sleeping six, who in turn suffered more lapses than subjects sleeping eight hours per night. The longer the subjects were sleep deprived, the more lapses they made. The number of lapses increased throughout the two-week study period. In fact, after ten days to two weeks of restricted sleep, research subjects progressively worsen to the point that they become as impaired as people who have been completely sleep deprived.

Research also reveals that people vary widely in response to sleep deprivation. Some people are profoundly affected, while others are more resistant to the impact of a single night of sleep loss but may, in turn, collapse after two sleepless nights. In general, most people can perform at fairly low levels when sleep-deprived and many can function well enough that their sleep deprivation is barely detectable.

Still, very few people are really immune to sleep deprivation. There seems to be a cognitive price for every minute of sleep less than the amount we need to be optimally alert. In one study, forty-eight subjects slept just four hour per night for two weeks. At the end of the two weeks, only one subject was able to perform as well as he had on day one, prior to sleep deprivation.

So is it worth it to pull an all-nighter before a test? Research indicates that it really depends on the type of test. For tests requiring rote memorization of simple facts, for example the presidents of the United States and their terms of office, studying all night may be beneficial because it involves the declarative memory system—the memory for facts. But for essay exams that involve making connections and analytical thinking, it's probably better to be well-rested because sleep deprivation sharply impairs critical thinking. It's a good idea to get ample sleep before math tests and other exams involving computation because evidence suggests that sleep deprivation creates a speed/accuracy trade-off on tasks involving cognitive throughput, such as mental arithmetic and digit substitution tasks. Sleep-deprived people are forced to slow down their cognitive operations in order to maintain accuracy.

LEARN WHILE YOU SLEEP?

You've probably seen ads for products claiming to help you learn, sharpen your memory, lose weight, and even break bad habits—all while you sleep. Is there anything to the premise that you can turn the seemingly wasted downtime of sleep into an opportunity to improve your self-esteem, learn a foreign language, drop extra pounds, enlarge your breasts, break an unhealthy addiction, or overcome your fear of public speaking?

The answer is a firm "maybe." It is certainly possible, for example, that reaffirming your intentions to eat healthily just before you go to sleep, and even listening to taped messages exhorting you to choose foods wisely may help to support your overall plan to lose weight. On the other hand, it's highly unlikely that you can become completely fluent in a foreign language without any study, simply by listening to tapes while you sleep. Seductive as the promise of subliminal learning—absorbing new material effortlessly while we sleep—may sound, sleep researchers explain that taped messages played while you sleep are of practically no value because the sound would have to wake you in order for learning to occur. This is because unlike hypnosis, a state in which many people are susceptible to spoken suggestion, during sleep, the brain is generally considered to be unresponsive to sensory input.

So why all the interest in hypnopaedia, the technical term for learning while sleeping? Probably because there is some experimental evidence that certain types of information can be reinforced during sleep. For example, in 1942 Lawrence LeShan tested whether sleep learning could influence behavior on boys attending summer camp. LeShan divided the boys into three groups. The first group consisted of twenty nail-biting boys, aged eight to twelve. There were two control groups: one with eight nail-biters, aged eight to ten; the other group had twelve nail biters, aged eleven to fourteen.

The first group listened to a recording while they slept that repeated, "My fingernails taste terribly bitter," three hundred times over the course of fifty-four consecutive nights. The other two groups did not hear any messages while they slept. LeShan found that 40 percent of the boys in the experimental group stopped biting their nails, which he interpreted as strong support for his hypothesis that listening to recorded messages during sleep can powerfully promote behavioral change.

A decade later, other researchers tested the theory that language could be taught during sleep. Using three groups of subjects, they attempted to teach Chinese to native English speakers. The first group listened to a recording while they slept that consisted of twenty-five Chinese words and their correct English translation, repeated fifteen times. The second group heard a recording of the same twenty-five Chinese words, repeated fifteen times, but the English translations they were given were incorrect. The third group served as a control group—they heard twenty-nine minutes of music while they slept.

The next morning, each group listened to the same recording that was played to the first group, and they were tested to assess their comprehension of the Chinese language. Since the first group performed better than the other two, the researchers concluded that learning can occur during sleep. More recent research has confirmed that reinforcement during sleep material already learned while awake may be beneficial. Rote memorization is the type of learning most likely to occur during sleep.

But the recent resurgence in excitement about sleep learning is probably the result of our increasingly pressured lives and our desire to make the most of every moment and to master the practice of multitasking. Couple this pressure to achieve with the promise of effortless learning and behavioral change, and it's easy to understand why so many of us fall prey to products assuring that we can improve our minds, bodies, and spirits while we sleep.

Recently, researchers discovered that scents can influence how sleep affects memory. Researchers had groups of subjects play a version of a concentration game, memorizing the location of card pairs on a computer screen. As they identified the location of each pair, the subjects received a burst of rose scent.

The subjects went to sleep about a half-hour later, wired with electrodes to monitor their deep–sleep activity, since that is when the brain processes newly acquired factual information most efficiently. The researchers also delivered bursts of the rose scent during this slow-wave sleep. Curiously, the scent did not wake the subjects or interrupt their sleep, and they reported no memory of it. Apparently, however, their brains perceived the scent, and preserved an almost perfect memory of the cards and their locations. The subjects scored an average of 97 percent on the card game, compared with 86 percent when they played the game and slept without exposure to the scent. The subjects did not receive the same benefit when they received bursts of scent just before sleep or during REM sleep rather than in deep sleep, and their improved scores were not attributable to practice or experience.

Research has revealed that specific regions of the cortex—the part of the brain involved in cognition, organization, and planning—communicate during deep sleep with the hippocampus, which records each day's memories. The studies assert that the cortex is telling the hippocampus to reactivate the same neurons that fired when a particular fact was learned. The hippocampus does this by encoding the firing sequence in the cortex necessary to consolidate memory.

The researchers also contend that olfactory sensing pathways in the brain lead more directly to the hippocampus than do visual and auditory ones. To confirm their suppositions, the researchers took MRI scans of the subjects' brains during their rose-scented sleep. As they predicted, regions of the cortex became noticeably more active with the scent than without, as did the hippocampus.

These findings imply that distinct sleep states may be specialized to integrate different kinds of learned information. For example, the researchers found that the rose scent did not improve memories of a learned finger-tapping sequence. This is because rhythmic memory does not appear to be consolidated by the hippocampus as are location and spatial orientation.

Mental Health and Emotional Well-being

There is no question that sleep deprivation has a profound effect on mood and mental health. And it's much more than waking up bleary-eyed or feeling grumpy or irritated. There is a strong association between sleep loss and depression, anxiety, and other mental health problems. It's not surprising that sleep deprivation affects mood and mental health when you consider that sleep involves a shift in the balance of the same neurotransmitters—serotonin, norepinephrine, dopamine, melatonin, and others—involved in governing cognition and emotional well-being.

There's also mounting evidence of a bidirectional relationship between sleep and health, especially mental health. Many studies have found that sleep disturbances contribute to the development of or increase the severity of various medical and psychiatric disorders, and these same disorders result in poor sleep quality—lending credence to the hypothesis that not only does poor or inadequate sleep affect health, but also that mental and physical health problems can affect the duration and quality of sleep.

Although the precise relationship between sleep and mental health has not yet been uncovered, one possible explanation is that conditions such as sleep apnea may contribute to mood disorders by depriving the brain of oxygen. Another way that sleep helps us to maintain optimal emotional and social functioning is by allowing the parts of the brain that control emotions and social interactions to rest while we sleep.

Sleep deprivation also may cloud moral judgment. Recent research found that following two sleepless nights, volunteer subjects displayed compromised ability to make decisions when presented with emotionally charged moral dilemmas.

The subjects were presented with a variety of scenarios and asked whether a given course of action would be appropriate or inappropriate. The situations ranged from minor, morally insignificant issues to serious personal dilemmas in which the subject's decision would harm someone in order to protect someone else.

The subjects were asked to assess the scenarios before and after fifty-three hours of sleep deprivation. The researchers found that the sleep-deprived subjects took more time to consider the more serious moral dilemmas, suggesting greater difficulty deciding upon a course of action when they were sleep-deprived than when they were well rested, but did not require additional time to evaluate the minor, morally insignificant scenarios.

Interestingly, some subjects changed their views of what was morally acceptable after they'd been awake for two days. The researchers observed, however, that subjects who had scored high in emotional intelligence were less susceptible to changes in moral judgments as a function of sleep loss.

The researchers speculate that their findings reflect the fact that sleep deprivation reduces metabolic activity in the ventromedial prefrontal cortex—the region of the brain that plays an important role in developing moral judgments. They also posit that sleep deprivation slows the brain's ability to synthesize cognitive and emotional information, which is how responses to serious moral dilemmas are formulated.

The Relationship Between Sleep and Sex

Conventional wisdom holds that participating in sexual activity promotes good, sound sleep and it is believed that sexual activity increases the need to sleep in many species. Among humans it is thought to induce sleep by inducing muscle relaxation, relieving stress and tension, and flooding the brain and body with the neurochemicals associated with pleasure, tranquility, and satisfaction. Anxieties and inhibitions tend to dissolve into feelings of emotional warmth, well being, and pleasant drowsiness.

Animal studies suggest that copulatory activity might be the source of neurohormonal processes that induce sleep and may involve the participation of gamma-aminobutyric acid (GABA), serotonin, or other neurohormonal regulators of sleep and wakefulness.

Interestingly, a recent study found that in men aged sixty-four to seventy-four years, the amount of nighttime sleep was associated with morning testosterone levels—there was a positive relationship between testosterone levels and sleep duration and quality in older healthy men. Previous research has found that androgen levels in healthy young men are highest on awakening and are reduced during sleep deprivation. Androgen levels quickly return to normal after regular sleep patterns resume.

Safety and Accidents

One of the scariest findings from sleep research laboratories is that reducing sleep time in healthy adults to between four and six hours per night produces cumulative increases in daytime performance deficits. These can become so severe that ultimately, they reach levels comparable to the deficits found under conditions of acute total sleep deprivation—all without the affected person feeling significantly sleepy. This finding, that sleep loss affects cognitive speed and accuracy, memory, and reaction time without the sleep-deprived person being aware of the deficits, suggests that the brain is vulnerable to chronically reduced sleep in a way that is not fully apparent in the subjective perception and assessment of sleepiness.

Workplace drowsiness is a recognized as a major cause of industrial and personal-injury accidents, compromised productivity, and even deaths. According to the National Sleep Foundation (NSF), the overwhelming majority of Americans believe that inadequate sleep impairs their work performance and puts them at increased risk for accidents, injuries, and health problems. The NSF estimates that sleep loss and workplace drowsiness cost U.S. industries at least $77 billion per year combined.

People who work in transportation services, public safety, health care, and the military, as well as the 17 percent of U.S. employees that work the night shift, are among the most perilously affected by sleep deprivation. Sleepiness accounts for one third of all fatal trucking accidents, and when a truck driver who has driven too many hours without rest dies in a crash, innocent people are usually also injured or killed. In 2003, 457,000 large trucks were involved in traffic crashes in the United States. The costs for fatal traffic accidents exceed $20 billion, including an estimated $8.7 billion in productivity losses, $2.5 billion in resource costs, and quality of life losses valued at $13.1 billion.

In February 2007, the National Transportation Safety Board told Congress that worker fatigue has been a probable cause of 40 percent of all train accidents and has been implicated in sixteen major train accidents during the past two decades. For train workers, the odds of experiencing an accident are high— workers can expect to be involved in a fatal railroad accident if they spend a working lifetime on the tracks.

The Federal Railroad Administration has asked Congress to repeal a one-hundred-year-old law that regulates workers' schedules, arguing that the laws do not reflect present-day scientific knowledge of the impact a lack of sleep has on transportation workers. Outdated rules governing the number of hours worked versus the number of hours of rest between shifts further compound the problem.

Currently, train crews and signal workers can work twelve hours straight with ten hours of rest. But when an employee works even one minute less than twelve hours, law mandates just eight hours of rest. Unpredictable schedules are also a problem. The Federal Railroad Administration advocates more rest between shifts, or shorter workdays.

Similarly, in the aviation industry, shift workers at risk of fatigue and sleep deprivation include pilots, cabin crew, maintenance engineers, air traffic controllers, and workers involved in the operation of aviation machinery. According to recent research, one of the highest sleep deprivation risks associated with those in aviation is the approach and landing phase of air travel.

This is especially important for those in the cockpit, who endure long, monotonous, mind-numbing periods of time that may lull them to drowsiness. Unlike other disciplines where the highest level of attention and concentration are required at the onset of the job or consistently throughout the shift, a flight crew must rise to peak performance at the final and most critical phase of the flight. Upon the approach to landing, they must suddenly regain wakefulness and heightened attentiveness in order to make critical landing decisions.

Lack of sleep increases the likelihood of making bad decisions during this critical phase: a fatigued pilot can have difficulty landing an aircraft, a sleep-deprived air traffic controller may incorrectly transmit critical instructions, an exhausted flight attendant or crew member may fail to communicate correctly, or an engineer may fit the wrong part. As a result, the U.S. Federal Aviation Administration (FAA) has mandated strict crew rest requirements to ensure adequate rest periods between flights.

Worker fatigue also has been named as a contributing factor in many of the most notorious incidents in recent history, including the 1979 Three Mile Island nuclear reactor meltdown, the 1986 nuclear accident at Chernobyl, the disastrous 1986 launch of the Space Shuttle Challenger, and the 11 million gallon oil spill caused when the oil tanker *Exxon Valdez* struck Bligh Reef in Prince William Sound, Alaska, in 1989.

The effect of sleep deprivation on automobile safety is a huge, underappreciated problem. Drowsy and distracted drivers may be deadly. More than half (60 percent) of adults who drive surveyed for the 2005 Sleep in America Poll reported that, within the past year, they had driven while feeling drowsy or sleepy. Scarier still, almost one-third of these survey respondents reported having had an accident or near accident at least once a month in the past. The same proportion said they had nodded off or fallen asleep while driving, even just for a brief moment. These kinds of lapses or microsleeps obviously pose a tremendous threat while driving. Even a lapse of several seconds could cause a driver to careen off the road, involuntarily change lanes or fail to stop at a stop sign or red light.

Drivers with untreated obstructive sleep apnea have been found to have as high an incidence of traffic accidents as drivers who are under the influence of alcohol. Drivers who have not had enough sleep can have driving problems that are comparable to those experienced by people with modest blood alcohol levels. The loss of as little as two to three hours of sleep affects an individual's ability to maintain a consistent speed and a stable road position.

The U.S. National Highway Traffic Safety Administration estimates that 100,000 motor vehicle accidents annually are the consequence of driver drowsiness or fatigue. Most motor vehicle and work-related accidents occur in the early to mid afternoon and in the very early morning hours. These are the times when sleep-deprived workers and drivers are least likely to be optimally alert.

Health-care workers also are at high risk for fatigue-related mishaps, accidents, and errors. According to the Institute of Medicine (IOM), sleep disorders and sleep deprivation are an unmet public health problem of major proportions. In a landmark report, the IOM, a division of the National Academies, found that as many as 98,000 deaths due to medical errors occur annually in U.S. hospitals.

Healthcare worker fatigue has a significant impact on patient safety and the quality of medical care patients receive. Many studies have confirmed the impact of fatigue on health-care personnel performance. One study of nursing fatigue suggests that it plays a role in increased error. For example, researchers found that nurses who worked a rotating schedule, when compared with nurses who predominantly worked day shifts, were more likely to fall asleep at work and get less sleep overall. These sleep-deprived nurses were nearly twice as likely to report making a medication error.

Hospitals operate around the clock, which necessitates shift work for many personnel. Physicians, especially those in training, typically work long hours and are often sleep-deprived. Medical residents work shifts as long as thirty hours—more consecutive hours than practically any other occupational group. In response to concerns about fatigue-related medical errors, the Accreditation Council for Graduate Medical Education (ACGME) instituted requirements in 2003 to limit the number of consecutive hours medical residents may work.

Happily, the effect of this rule was felt very soon after it was enacted. Research reported by the National Institute of Occupational Safety and Health (NIOSH) found that the rate of serious medical errors committed by first-year doctors in training in two intensive care units at a Boston hospital fell significantly when traditional thirty-hours-in-a-row extended work shifts were eliminated and when the first-year physicians' continuous work schedule was limited to sixteen hours.

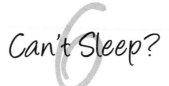

Can't Sleep?

A flock of sheep that leisurely pass by
One after one; the sound of rain, and bees
Murmuring; the fall of rivers, winds and seas,
Smooth fields, white sheets of water, and pure sky;
I've thought of all by turns, and still I lie
Sleepless . . .
                                —William Wordsworth, "To Sleep"

Nearly everyone has experienced an occasional problem getting to sleep or staying asleep. Problems falling asleep may be caused by stress or anxiety—an argument with a coworker, disagreement with a spouse, or a looming deadline at work or school, or the stress of experiences and worries far more serious. Pain or discomfort also may prevent you from falling asleep easily, especially if you can't sleep in your usual position or can't find a comfortable position. Eating or drinking, especially caffeine or alcohol, too close to your bedtime can disrupt normal sleep patterns as can nicotine and other drugs. Even exercising late in the day may make it harder to fall asleep.

Practice Good Sleep Hygiene

Sleep hygiene refers to how well one sleeps. It's also the term used to describe the conditions, habits, and practices that promote continuous and restorative sleep, including establishing regular bedtimes and waking times, allowing adequate time for sleep, restricting activities at bedtime that do not promote sleep, and modifying environmental factors so that they enhance, rather than impede, restful sleep.

Here are some simple steps you can take to improve your sleep hygiene. Some of them are simply good, old-fashioned common sense, but others may surprise you.

Diet

In general, it is unwise to eat in the four hours before you're planning to go to sleep. Late dinners and midnight snacks busy the body with the biochemistry and physical actions of digestion, which are hardly conducive to sound sleep. It also may help to avoid spicy, fried, and fatty foods, and mint, all of which may increase acid reflux and disrupt sleep.

If you're hungry at bedtime and must eat, try a light snack like milk and some crackers or a cup of caffeine-free herbal tea and a slice of whole-grain toast. Milk and other dairy products are good choices because they contain tryptophan, an essential amino acid that promotes sleep. Other good choices for late-night snacks include small portions of turkey or chicken or whole-grain cereal with milk and a banana.

Avoid caffeine and other stimulants (including cola, coffee, cocoa, nicotine, and prescription and over-the-counter drugs such as Anacin and Excedrin that contain caffeine) and alcohol in the six hours before bedtime. While it's true that alcohol may make you feel drowsy and can help you fall asleep more readily, it also acts to disrupt the sleep cycle, making it less likely that you'll wake feeling refreshed.

Environment

The ideal environment for sleep is a comfortable bed in a dark, quiet, and relatively cool room. A sleeping temperature of 60 to 65 degrees is ideal for most people, even in cold weather. In the summer, use a quiet fan to circulate air, or an air-conditioner set at about 70 degrees.

It may be helpful to view the bed and bedroom as a kind of soothing sleep sanctuary and to avoid other activities in the space designated for sleeping. Basically, your bedroom should be used exclusively for relaxation, sleep, and sex. For example, it is wise to avoid turning your bed into a home office by working on a laptop, paying bills, or talking on the phone in bed. Don't watch television, eat, or argue in bed. In other words, try to avoid bringing the sounds and stresses of your work, family life, or relationships to bed with you.

Don't place the telephone at your bedside, or if the phone must be there, turn off the ringer when you go to sleep. Similarly, for many troubled sleepers, it's helpful to move the clock out of sight and hearing distance—loud ticking can keep you awake, and watching minutes and hours elapse when you're trying to get to sleep may only heighten feelings of time pressure and anxiety. Setting an alarm clock for your scheduled arise time and then placing it on a shelf or dresser out of view can help to prevent anxiety-fueled clock watching.

If street noise, loud neighbors, or a snoring partner prevent you from falling asleep or staying asleep, then you may want to invest in earplugs, a white noise machine, or a fan that hums to block out the unwanted sounds. Similarly, if light is a problem, try dark shades on bedroom windows or a sleep mask that covers your eyes completely.

If you find yourself unable to fall asleep within twenty minutes of getting into bed or if you wake during the night and cannot fall back to sleep shortly, then you should get up, leave your bedroom, and engage in a quiet activity elsewhere. Try not to fall asleep outside your bedroom. Return to bed when and only when you are sleepy. Repeat this process as often as necessary throughout the night.

Alone or Together?

According to the National Sleep Foundation, more than half of Americans (61 percent) share their beds with significant others. For some, sharing a bed is a source of comfort and a way to achieve intimacy and freedom from the distractions of the day together. But for others, adjusting to sharing a bed is not without conflict. Disagreements arise about bedroom temperature, the position of the bed, which side each partner prefers, how to make the bed, sheet and blanket stealing, having a television in the bedroom, reading and eating in bed, and even the appropriate attire, if any, for sleep. Couples also disagreed about the location and sound of alarm clocks and whether to allow children or pets into the bed.

When one member of a sleeping couple snores or suffers from insomnia, the other may unintentionally "catch" the sleep problem as a result of being awakened often throughout the night. So while most couples prefer to sleep together, there are times when it makes sense, and may even be preferable, to sleep separately. For example, many menopausal women suffer hot flashes at night and prefer very cool sleeping quarters and just a sheet covering them, even in cold winter months. When their sleep partners are unable to make do with extra blankets, then it may be time for temporary relocation. Similarly, older men suffering from benign enlargement of the prostate gland may rise frequently during the night to use the bathroom. If their departures and returns to bed disrupt their partners' sleep, then sleeping apart may be a better option than chronic sleep deprivation.

Although it's certainly not a how-to book for sleeping with a partner suffering from sleep problems, Paul Rosenblatt's book *Two in a Bed: The Social System of Couple Bed Sharing* (State University of New York Press, 2006) does offer insight into how sleeping together affects a couple's relationship. Rosenblatt interviewed more than forty bed-sharing couples and queried them about a variety of sleep-related issues, including winding down and waking up, cold feet and tucked sheets, who sleeps near the door and who gets pushed to the edge, snoring, spooning, sleep talking, sleep walking, and other behaviors we continuously negotiate in falling asleep, staying asleep, and waking up each morning beside a partner. Rosenblatt contends that sleep should no longer be viewed solely as an individual phenomenon, since for most Americans it is not.

Increasingly, couples appear to be opting for separate bedrooms. A February 2007 survey conducted by the National Association of Home Builders found that builders and architects forecast that more than half of all custom homes would feature dual master suites by 2015. Demand is increasing for separate sleep sanctuaries and even small rooms off of master bedroom suites where snorers or night owls can be banished to permit their partners to sleep without interruptions.

EXERCISE

Regular physical exercise during the day is associated with sound, healthy sleep, but you should exercise well before you plan to go to bed, since vigorous or even moderate exercise may serve to rev you up rather than help you unwind in anticipation of sleep.

SCHEDULE

Going to bed and waking at the same time everyday is an important aspect of sleep hygiene. Tempting as it may be to stay up very late and sleep in until noon on weekends, it will make it very difficult for you to get back on track on Monday. Be certain to schedule enough time for sleep—feeling pressured to fall asleep quickly because you only have six hours allotted for sleep will not help you to get to sleep easily. In general, it's helpful to plan enough time so that you can devote time to relaxing before bed and sleeping for seven to eight hours.

It's also a good idea to develop pre-sleep rituals to help you to wind down and decompress from your day. Children's sleep improves with pre-sleep rituals like a bath, lullaby, and story, and adults can reap the same benefits. Adults can add gentle relaxation exercises like meditation, deep breathing, and some of the other stress-management techniques we'll describe later on to help calm and quiet the mind and body before sleep.

If possible, wake up to sunlight or very bright lights in the morning. Sunlight helps the body's internal biological clock reset itself each day. Sleep experts recommend exposure to an hour of morning sunlight for people having problems falling asleep.

LIMIT NAPS

Avoid taking long naps during the day. Napping in the late afternoon or early evening can disrupt nighttime sleep. Not all napping is bad—in fact, recent research reveals that brief midday naps can help office workers, especially men, reduce their risk of heart disease. Researchers believe that naps might benefit the heart by offering brief relief from work-related stress. The researchers concluded that, "An afternoon siesta in a healthy individual may act as a stress-reducing habit, and there is considerable evidence that stress has both short- and long-term adverse effects on the incidence of, and mortality from, coronary heart disease."

In fact, the news about the relationship between napping and heart health so impressed French health minister Xavier Bertrand that in early 2007 he called for research to determine whether French workers should be allowed to nap on the job. Despite their relatively light workload compared to their American counterparts—French workers average thirty-five-hour work weeks and enjoy ample vacation and time off—more than half of French workers (56 percent) contend that poor sleep has a negative impact on their job performance and productivity. The government also attributes as much as 30 percent of highway accidents in the country to sleepiness.

In response to these concerns, the French government recently announced a $9 million campaign to improve public awareness about sleep problems, and France's state-run health insurance provider has sent letters publicizing the importance of good sleep. The French Health Ministry's Web site, "Passport to Sleep," provides practical information about how to ensure quality sleep. It advises reducing consumption of coffee, tea, colas, and exercise after 8 p.m., eschewing television and working late into the evening, and tuning in to the body's natural sleep signals, such as yawning.

Some offices and manufacturing plants in the United States encourage on-the-job naps, reporting that napping improves employee performance by boosting productivity and reducing errors and work-site accidents. Another emerging trend is sleep salons—places where people can go to nap, for a price. At Yelo, a Manhattan sleep salon, patrons can rent a hexagonal-shaped private chamber for naps ranging in length from twenty to forty minutes. Each chamber is furnished with a beige leather recliner and a blanket of Nepalese cashmere and features low lighting and a sleep-inducing soundtrack. Many spas offer aromatherapy and lavender oil massages aimed at enhancing sleep.

Manage Stress and Anxiety

Many people complain that as soon as they lie down to sleep, they replay the stressful events of their day, anticipate the demands of the next day, or worry about ongoing problems. This may be because it's the first quiet moment they've had all day and the first opportunity to consider troubling events or issues. So, it may be helpful to schedule worrying earlier in the day, during a designated worry period, in which you actually commit your concerns to paper and devote a few minutes to considering them and formulating solutions to them. It is vitally important that you write your worry list and devote worrying time outside the bedroom, and that you schedule it well before bedtime.

In the next section, we'll look at a variety of ways to relieve and manage stress that may be interfering with your ability to sleep.

Coming to Grips with Stress

The time to relax is when you don't have time for it.
—Sydney J. Harris, American journalist

WHAT YOUR DOCTOR CAN DO
TO HELP YOU COPE WITH STRESS

There are definitely times when the influences of stress are so severe that medical intervention may be appropriate. Stress can actually damage the limbic organs of the brain and the constant hypervigilance of an overstimulated sympathetic nervous system can deplete the adrenal glands as well as a broad spectrum of nutrients, enzymes, minerals, and metabolic cofactors.

In such situations, it may well be advisable to consult with a medical practitioner. You and your physician may explore a number of different stress-management options, including pharmaceutical drugs for the treatment of some aspects of stress such as chronic anxiety or depression, depending on your individual situation. While these drugs may be extremely important, even life-saving interventions, it's important to remember that in most cases they don't actually solve the problems of stress at their root causes. It may be tempting to engineer a life in which drugs are used to mask the effects of stress, but a healthy life depends, ultimately, upon transformation, not simply management of symptoms. In recognition of this fact, more and more health-care practitioners are starting to use drug therapies as temporary, transitional tools as they help their patients to obtain other forms of support.

A variety of publicly available resources exist to help people learn about stress and stress management. The American Psychological Association maintains an excellent Web site with health education and information on a variety of important topics, including stress. Another excellent online resource is the Web site of the American Institute of Stress. The AIS site contains information and articles about the health impact and treatment of stress. You can find the APA section on stress at http://www.apa.org/topics/topicstress.html. The American Institute of Stress is online at http://www.stress.org.

What Your Doctor Can Do to Help You Sleep Better

When sleep problems persist beyond a few nights or are having a serious impact on your ability to enjoy life, then it's time to consult with your physician. As we've seen, sleep problems may be attributable to a host of medical conditions, such as obstructive sleep apnea, that are easily diagnosed and treated.

Your physician may order an overnight sleep study to assess whether physical, mechanical problems or neurological disorders are interfering with your sleep. Most sleep studies also involve a complete physical examination and an assessment of sleep hygiene.

If you suffer from allergies, be certain to mention your allergies during the visit to your doctor about sleep problems. Your allergies may be causing or contributing to sleep problems. A year-long study of people suffering from allergic rhinitis found that this condition impaired all dimensions of sleep. Compared to members of a control group, study subjects experienced more daytime fatigue and sleepiness as well as impaired memory, mood, and sleep quality.

PRESCRIPTION SLEEP MEDICATIONS

Americans are popping more sleeping pills than ever before. About 42 million sleeping pill prescriptions were filled in 2005, and during 2006 U.S. sales of prescription sleeping medications reached $3.7 billion.

Prescription sleep medications are meant to provide temporary relief from insomnia, which is not a long-term solution. Some researchers and physicians are concerned that theses sedative-hypnotic drugs are being prescribed too freely and are used for too long, especially because very little is known about the consequences of long-term use. Others are concerned about the proliferation of direct-to-consumer advertising of these drugs. Pharmaceutical manufacturers spent more than $300 million in 2006 to persuade troubled sleepers that their products were safe and effective. The research firm TNS Media Intelligence reported that in 2005 and 2006, Sanofi-Aventis spent a total of nearly $350 million to advertise Ambien and Ambien CR. Sepracor spent more than $500 million on advertising for Lunesta during that same two-year period. And Takeda, the maker of Rozerem, spent about $100 million.

Nearly everyone has seen the luminous luna moth fluttering over the bed of a blissful sleeper who has taken Lunesta. Who could forget the recent television ads for ramelteon (Rozerem, a prescription drug for insomnia) that featured a dream sequence that included a man having a conversation with Abraham Lincoln and a talking beaver?

Historically, prescription sleep aids were largely barbiturates like phenobarbital and benzodiazepines such as Halcion, which carried a strong risk of dependence and addiction, so their use was generally short term. Newer, short-acting sedative-hypnotics cause you to feel sleepy by increasing the normal effects of the brain chemical gamma-aminobutyric acid (GABA). They are more effective and safer for long-term, nightly use than benzodiazepines but still have some risk of dependency. Although the newer drugs—Ambien, Lunesta, Rozerem, Sonata, and others—are not believed to carry the same risk of dependence as older drugs like benzodiazepines, which work by slowing down the central nervous system to cause drowsiness, some researchers and drug users have reported what is called the "next-day" effect, a continued sleepiness hours after awakening from a drug-induced slumber. Along with daytime sleepiness following drug-induced sleep, some users also experience a kind of amnesia when they resume their usual daytime activities too quickly after taking the drugs.

There also have been worrisome reports of users of the popular sleeping pill Ambien sleepwalking, sleep driving, preparing food and eating it, and even making phone calls while asleep, then not remembering any of it. In rare instances there have been cases of dangerous, potentially life-threatening reactions called anaphylaxis (an immediate, severe allergic respiratory difficulty and drop in blood pressure that may cause fainting, collapse, or loss of consciousness).

As a result of these side effects, in March 2007 the U.S. Food and Drug Administration (FDA) called for label changes on these drugs that provide stronger warnings about possible side effects. The warnings also include information about rare risk of life-threatening allergic reactions to sleep medications. There have been recent reports of patients experiencing allergic reactions in which the air passages or face swells up after using one of the newest drugs on the market, Rozerem. The FDA also advised long-term follow-up studies to determine how frequently side effects and adverse reactions occur, especially sleep-driving, sleep-eating, and other unusual activities.

A few short weeks after the FDA called for revised safety warnings for sleeping pills, Merck, a leading pharmaceutical company announced that it was halting development of a product in progress—gabadoxol, a sleeping pill the company had previously touted as a potential blockbuster. Development of the drug was canceled because it not only failed a trial of its efficacy but also because serious side-effects, including hallucinations and disorientation, emerged during clinical trials.

OVER-THE-COUNTER SLEEP MEDICATIONS

Like prescription sleep aids, over-the-counter (OTC) sleep medications are not intended for long-term use. The principal ingredient of most over-the-counter sleeping pills is an antihistamine. Antihistamines are generally taken to relieve allergy symptoms, but they also make you feel very sleepy. Common nonprescription sleep medications are Sleep-Eze, Sominex, Nytol, and Unisom, which contain antihistamines such as diphenhydramine hydrochloride, diphenhydramine citrate, or doxylamine succinate. Some OTC sleep aids contain both an antihistamine and a pain reliever.

Just because you can purchase them without a prescription does not mean that over-the-counter sleeping pills are harmless. In fact, they may produce a range of side effects, some of which are comparable to those of their prescription counterparts. Common side-effects of nonprescription sleep aids include drowsiness the day after use, dizziness, fatigue, headaches, reduced alertness, vomiting, mild memory impairment, problems with coordination or balance, constipation, urinary retention, blurred vision, and dry mouth and throat. It's also easy to develop a tolerance for over-the-counter sleep medications after a few days of use. Many users quickly discover that they need higher doses to feel drowsy enough to sleep.

According to the American Academy of Sleep Medicine (AASM), a professional organization dedicated to the assurance of quality care for patients with sleep disorders, the use of OTC sleep aids is common. In one survey of 2,181 adults, more than 10 percent of adults said that they used an OTC sleep aid in the past year. Another survey found that 21.4 percent of people with daytime problems resulting from insomnia take an OTC medication to help them sleep. The official AASM position on OTC sleep medications is that "[s]ufficient evidence does not exist to support over-the-counter (OTC) sleep aids as an effective treatment for insomnia. OTC sleep aids that contain antihistamine may provide modest, short-term benefits for adults with mild cases of insomnia. It is important to be aware, however, that the use of antihistamines may produce a variety of side effects."

COGNITIVE BEHAVIORAL THERAPY

Many sleep researchers and therapists feel that a brief form of psychotherapy called cognitive behavioral therapy (CBT) can help insomniacs and others with disordered sleep regain quality sleep without resorting to drugs. CBT is based on the premise that thinking influences emotions and behavior—that feelings and actions originate with thoughts. So if clients experience unwanted feelings and behaviors, it is important for them to identify the thinking that causes the feelings and behaviors and learn how to replace their dysfunctional thoughts with thoughts that produce more desirable reactions. CBT posits that it is possible to change the way people feel and act, even if their circumstances do not change. Using CBT, clients reorganize their thinking about sleep, which is often based on incorrect assumptions, and learn to change counterproductive aspects of their sleep hygiene.

CBT teaches the advantages of feeling, at worst, calm when faced with undesirable situations. Clients learn that they will confront undesirable events, such as sleepless nights or difficulty falling or staying asleep, whether they become troubled about them or not. When they are troubled about sleep disturbances, then they have two problems—the sleep disturbance, and the troubling feelings about the sleep disturbance. Clients learn that when they do not become troubled about disrupted sleep and sleep deprivation they can reduce the number of problems they face by half.

CBT is a relatively fast-acting, structured, and directed treatment modality. It is short-term, with clients receiving an average of just sixteen sessions. In contrast to other forms of therapy, CB therapists tend to offer more instruction than practitioners of other forms of therapy and usually assign homework in the form of reading assignments and practicing the techniques learned.

Unlike other therapies in which the therapist-client relationship is central to the process, CBT emphasizes an active, collaborative, client-directed process in which clients learn rational self-counseling skills. Cognitive-behavioral therapists aim to understand what their clients want out of life and then help their clients achieve those objectives. Since CBT is based on an educational model and the assumption that most emotional and behavioral reactions are learned, therapists serve as teachers—they question, listen, instruct, encourage their clients to question themselves, and support clients' progress. In turn clients become students of life as they learn and implement the action, behaviors, and sleep strategies they have learned.

The National Association of Cognitive-Behavioral Therapists (NACBT) emphasizes that CBT is much more than "just talking" and that the educational emphasis and reliance on rational thinking as opposed to assumptions enable clients to achieve lasting, long-term results. The professional association asserts that, "When people understand how and why they are doing well, they can continue doing what they are doing to make themselves well. Should insomnia recur after CBT ends, clients have the tools and strategies to improve their sleep hygiene on their own."

What You Can Do About Stress

Do not anticipate trouble or worry about what may never happen. Keep in the sunlight.
                                        —Benjamin Franklin

One of the most exciting things about stress reduction is that there are so many things you can do to support your own healing and relieve troubling symptoms. Many of these techniques are free, or nearly so. Some, like a few of the bodywork techniques, require assistance, but the majority can be done on your own.

What most techniques of stress reduction have in common is that they work, on some level, to help cool down the chronic overactivation of the sympathetic trunk of the nervous system. Remember that when the sympathetic side of the nervous system is overstimulated—that is, when the body's "gas pedal" is always floored—it becomes very difficult for those functions that work with parasympathetic signals, the body's "brake pedal," to work properly.

Along with digestion and assimilation, parasympathetic responses are critical for rest, relaxation, sleep, healthy breathing, and even sexual arousal. And while we usually think of relaxation as a passive process—the absence of stimulation—it's more correct to conceive of unwinding as an active process that requires the stimulation of the parasympathetic nervous system. Clearly, activities that help to shift the balance from sympathetic to parasympathetic will not only help us to relax but also to access the physical systems needed for restoration and healing, and even for creative thinking and self-expression.

COMPLEMENTARY AND ALTERNATIVE THERAPIES

Complementary and alternative medicine (CAM) therapies are generally defined as medical practices that are as yet unproven by conventional Western science and not presently considered an integral part of conventional medicine. According to the 2002 National Health Interview Survey more than 1.6 million civilian adults in the United States used CAM therapies and practices to treat insomnia or trouble sleeping. Since in many instances, people can obtain CAM treatments themselves, without seeing a health-care provider, making an accurate estimate of the prevalence of CAM treatment for insomnia is challenging.

Analysis of the survey data revealed that younger respondents and those with higher education were more likely to use CAM therapies to treat insomnia or trouble sleeping. The survey also found that insomnia or trouble sleeping was most strongly linked with one of four health conditions—hypertension, congestive heart failure, anxiety or depression, and obesity.

While nearly two-thirds of those surveyed employed biologically based therapies (herbs, nutrients, supplements), almost a third tried mind-body therapies (biofeedback, meditation, relaxation) and less than 10 percent used alternative medical systems (traditional Chinese medicine, Ayurvedic medicine) or manipulative and body based therapies (massage, yoga). More than 60 percent of subjects said they had combined CAM practices with traditional treatment for sleep disorders, and about 40 percent said they had turned to CAM practices when conventional treatments failed to help them. The survey also found that a whopping 60.7 percent of respondents told conventional medical practitioners that they were using a CAM therapy for insomnia or trouble sleeping—a much higher proportion than reported in previous surveys about CAM use. The National Center For Complementary and Alternative Medicine (NCCAM) is one of the National Institutes of Health. NCCAM is actively supporting research about whether CAM therapies are effective for sleep disorders. Examples of NCCAM research studies include:

• An assessment of whether the herb valerian will help healthy older adults with sleep disorders is underway at the University of Washington.

• At Brigham and Women's Hospital in Boston, investigators are looking at a program of relaxation and yoga as treatment for insomnia. Another study at the same institution is seeking to determine if vitamin B12 may be an effective treatment for a form of delayed sleep phase syndrome that affects blind people.

- University of Chicago researchers are examining the action of hops, an herb that has been used alone and in combination with valerian for sleep problems.

- Investigators at the University of Pennsylvania are comparing low doses of melatonin, high doses of melatonin, and a placebo in older adults with low levels of natural melatonin to see if any of these therapies improves sleep quality.

- University of North Carolina researchers are trying to find out whether high-intensity light could help treat problems such as sleep/wake disorders, depressive symptoms, agitation, and other behavioral issues that afflict persons afflicted with Alzheimer's disease (a progressive, neurodegenerative disease characterized by loss of function and death of nerve cells in several areas of the brain, leading to loss of mental functions such as memory and learning. It is the most common cause of dementia).

- Harvard University researchers are studying the effects of blue light therapy on sleep cycles.

- University of Arizona investigators are evaluating the effect of homeopathic remedies on sleep patterns. (Homeopathic remedies are based on the idea that substances that produce symptoms of sickness in healthy people will have a curative effect when given in very dilute quantities to sick people who exhibit those same symptoms. Homeopathic remedies are believed to stimulate the body's own healing processes.)

Stress Busters

> *There must be quite a few things that a hot bath won't*
> *cure, but I don't know many of them.*
>
> —Sylvia Plath, *The Bell Jar*

There are many ways to help control and reduce our experience of stress. In the following sections, we're going to look in some detail at meditation, the craniosacral stillpoint, and helpful nutritional supplements that encourage natural relaxation and relief from stress. You can relieve many symptoms of stress by using the following:

- **Simple meditation exercises**, such as following the breath, and more involved meditations, such as guided journeys through your own body.

- **Craniosacral stillpoint induction**, an amazingly simple technique that breaks up stuck stress patterns in the nervous system and presses a kind of "reset button."

- **Nutritional supplements** that encourage the body to balance and unwind in a natural, harmonious way.

- **Basic movement therapy**, including classic floor exercises.

It's also important to take steps to build your resiliency to stress by:

- Scheduling **regular exercise**—walk, bike, play a sport, work out at the gym—anything that gets you up and moving.

- Getting **bodywork** such as massage or other forms of therapeutic touch.

- *Seeking* out **support groups in your community**—local hospitals or clinics frequently offer classes that deal with stress reduction in general, or specific techniques like yoga, tai chi, aerobic exercise, or nutritional counseling.

- Making space in your life for your **hobbies and interests**, even if they seem at first like a luxury or indulgence. Investing in your own fulfillment is the best way to be strong and resilient for others who depend upon you.

- Becoming involved in fulfilling **social and civic activities**, such as community or charity work.

SOCIAL CONNECTEDNESS

Family, friends, active interests, and community involvement may do more than simply help people enjoy their lives. Social activities and relationships may actually enable people to live longer by preventing or delaying development of many diseases by supporting emotional resiliency, which in turn helps to prevent the deleterious effects of stress. During the past three decades, research has demonstrated that social experiences, activities, interpersonal relationships, and work stress are related to health, well-being, and longevity. The kind of work stress that causes the greatest harm to physical and mental health is effort-reward imbalance—when great effort is made and the effort is neither recognized nor rewarded. Studies have found that women appear more vulnerable to job stress, while men's health seems more dependent on the availability of social relationships and emotional support.

A SIMPLE MEDITATION—FOLLOWING YOUR BREATH

Historically, meditation has been used to enhance spiritual

growth and in religious training and practices, but it also is a powerful self-care measure that may be used to relieve stress and promote relaxation. Transcendental meditation, an Indian practice that involves sitting and silently chanting a mantra—a word repeated to quiet the mind—aims to produce a healthy state of relaxation.

During the 1960s, Dr. Herbert Benson studied meditation, and he and his colleagues at Harvard University Medical School showed that by meditating, people could reduce heart and respiration rates, lower blood levels of the hormone cortisol, and increase alpha waves in the brain. Dr. Benson developed a relaxation technique loosely based on transcendental meditation that he called the "relaxation response," and this technique quickly gained recognition in the United States and Europe.

Although meditation has been a part of countless spiritual and religious traditions for thousands of years, the act of meditation itself is free of any particular belief system or theology. The goal in meditation is to allow the mind and body to settle into a natural state of relaxed awareness. This is not a dream state, or a sleep state, or a state of reflective, intellectual thought. Rather, the meditative state is one in which you remain aware of your surroundings but you do not use your mind to judge or interpret. Instead of projecting ourselves out into the world, meditation is a time when we simply breathe the world in, exactly as it is.

There is an old story about a young man in India who asks a famous spiritual master for instruction in meditation. "That's easy," says the master. "Just sit on this cushion for an hour and don't think about monkeys."

Of course, as soon as the mind is given the instruction to "not think," we tend to think about not thinking. Then we think about what we would be thinking if we *were* thinking, which, of course, is thinking. It's like walking between two mirrors. We don't see two reflections of ourselves—we see an infinite number.

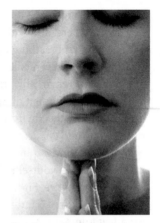

The goal of meditation is not to apply a rule to suppress thought but rather, to train ourselves *not to follow* our thoughts—to allow them to arise, as they naturally will, but then to float away like bubbles. We tend to attach our thoughts together, like the cars of a train, one following the next,

Regular meditation can help improve the quality of sleep.

each thought triggering and attaching to the next. In meditation, we simply allow everything to be as it is, without judgment or commentary, both in the outer world unfolding around us, and in our inner world as well.

As simple as it sounds, it takes some doing. Especially in the modern world, with telephones and television and computers and radios and MP3 players and honking horns and police sirens . . . we seldom have a moment of true quiet. Our nervous systems adapt to this constant onslaught of signals by screening out the top level of our awareness of them, but we cannot screen out the constant stress created in the nervous system. Meditation is a unique time in which to do that, and the result is a quieting of the mind that allows the nervous system the chance to settle down and a time for feelings, emotions, creative inspirations, and other treasures of the heart to arise.

Many books have been written on meditation, but the

simplest form of meditation is following the breath, which you can do anywhere, at any time. Unless it becomes problematic, like the labored breathing experienced by people with asthma, emphysema, or severe allergies, we tend to take breathing for granted. But, remarkably, from the first moments after we're born until the moment of our death, we are literally connected to life through the rhythm of our breath. This is a profound relationship and an ideal focal point for meditation.

If you can, find a quiet place. If you can't find a quiet place, make one inside yourself. This may be hard at first but it gets easier with practice. Sit in a comfortable position—no special posture is required. Find a way to sit where you can be relaxed for a few minutes without cramping up—on a chair or on the floor. If you have to lie down, avoid the temptation to fall asleep or to nod off into a twilight state. On the other hand, if the quality of your sleep has been poor, the first few times you try this your body may decide that you need the deeper relaxation of sleep more than you need meditation.

Allow your eyes to become unfocused, resting your gaze several feet in front of your body. Take a slow, peaceful breath in and put all your awareness on the breath itself. Feel how it moves through your nostrils. Feel your chest expand. Stay with the sensory aspects of the breath—nothing else. Exhale comfortably, preferably through your mouth, and again, notice the sensations of your breath. Allow the breath to simply flow out of your body, and then breathe in again.

As you do this, breathing in and out, staying focused on the movement of the breath and on sensations, your thoughts will naturally fall away. If a thought arises, don't fight it. Trying to suppress a thought is like stepping between two mirrors. Simply don't follow the thought. Allow it to float away. If another thought arises, notice as it passes and stay focused on your breathing.

Most people, after an initial period where many thoughts tend to arise, quickly fall into a peaceful rhythm, breathing in and out, lulled by the gentle sensations of air making a braid, spiraling into the nose, down the lungs, and out the mouth. You may find this so refreshing that after just a few minutes you feel recharged. Again, others may initially feel tired, indicating that their bodies need a chance to rest.

A Personally Guided Tour

If you like this simple meditation, you can find any number of books and Web sites that help you move into more involved techniques, including guided meditations. These are imaginary journeys that are conducted, though verbal suggestions, by a guide. There are tapes and CDs with guided meditation experiences, and you can also make up your own. A good guided meditation does not tell you where to go or what to see with your inner eye but rather tells a story that suggests what to look for and where to focus your awareness. Your own psyche will supply the images that are most meaningful for you.

While this may sound naïve, remember that many parts of your brain and nervous system—especially the limbic system where primary stress responses originate and often get stuck— do not draw a strong distinction between physical stimuli from the outer world and imaginary stimuli from our interior world. All forms of meditation and guided imagery exploit this fact and the body obligingly follows. If you have a part of the body that hurts or has a hard time healing—anything from an ache in your head to a twisted ankle to poor digestion—you can invent your own guided meditations.

Start by lying down with your eyes closed. This is a different type of meditation from breath following and has a different aim; it is more like achieving a consciously induced dream state. Use breath following to calm your system and then put all your awareness into your feet. Allow yourself to feel your feet—your toes, the tops of your feet, the soles—and simply focus on the sensations, as you did earlier with your breath. You are not trying to understand or change or fix anything. Instead, you are shifting your awareness so that you become totally immersed in the reality of your own body.

Next, allow your awareness to travel from your feet up into your ankles, calves, and the lower parts of your legs. Stay immersed in your body—without thinking or judging. Focus only on sensations, noting what you feel, and then move further up, into your knees, then your thighs, staying completely at the level of noticing feelings without having to do anything about them.

Continue in this way through the core of your body. Move slowly enough so that each part of the body has a chance to speak to you. We normally don't listen to our bodies except when they tell us we're hungry or tired or have to go to the bathroom. We normally allow the language our bodies speak to be heard and interpreted only by our autonomic nervous systems and endocrine responses. But in this process, we are allowing ourselves to hear our bodies speaking to us. It's not a language we understand in words and ideas—it's a language spoken entirely in feelings.

When you get to your heart, spend a little extra time. The heart is the functional center of the body. Every other part of the body talks with the heart. At this point, some people experience enormous emotional responses, but there is no reason or need to express these feelings in words. Simply allow the feelings to arise, the way in breathing we allowed thoughts to arise, without the need to grasp and understand them.

When you're ready, continue to move the focus of your awareness, up through the chest, and the neck, along your face and through your head. Don't stop at the top of the head—continue this process to a point about six inches above your head—outside of the skull.

Once you've tracked your awareness through your entire body, allow your awareness to settle into the place that you want to work on —the place that hurts, or is stuck, or is the site of illness. Again, don't try to understand or judge or interpret. Simply become profoundly present at that location and listen with your inner ears. Be content with being still—this is one of the greatest services you can do to your body: being still and listening. Places that are ill, that are hurt, have not been able to get through to the rest of the body to find the support they need to grow and regenerate properly. This is an important moment—consciously reaching out to a hurt place and allowing it to speak its needs.

When you have a sensation in this part of the body—even if you don't recognize or understand the sensation at all—imagine the pathway through your body from the place you are focusing on to your heart. In your inner awareness, feel a movement, like a trickling stream, between this place and your heart. Feel the hurt place flowing to the heart and, after a time, an answering flow from the heart back to the hurt place. Allow this flow to run for as long as it's comfortable. At some point, the flow will either stop, or you will no longer feel interested in focusing on it. This is a natural signal to stop.

Once again, put your awareness into the place above your head and slowly move your point of focus down through your body, stopping only where you are moved to stop, listening whenever some place in your body feels like it has something to say. Continue until your awareness arrives back in your feet, especially the soles of your feet. Take a few slow, conscious breaths and open your eyes. Wait a few minutes before standing up or trying to walk. This can be an extraordinarily powerful meditation. It can access your "inner physician," the part of your psyche that knows more about your body and your own personal situation than anyone else.

The Point of Stillness

Craniosacral therapy is a sophisticated bodywork technique that works with the deep physiological rhythm of the brain and nervous system. Just like the more obvious rhythms of our breath and our heartbeat, but at a slower, more subtle level, the reservoir of fluid that surrounds the brain and the spinal chord also breathes, about six to ten times every minute. During this time, there is an expansion phase during which the volume and pressure of cerebrospinal fluid increases, followed by a contraction phase in which the fluid volume decreases.

But the craniosacral rhythm does much more than circulate fluid around the brain. The rhythm also acts like a kind of internal sonar, providing a deep pulse around which many other parts of the body organize and communicate. In fact, a skilled practitioner of craniosacral therapy can feel the minute reflections of this core rhythm in every other part of the body, even as far away from the skull as you can get—in the toes and ankles.

Dr. Jonathan Upledger, the osteopathic physician who developed many of the techniques of craniosacral therapy, discovered that the craniosacral rhythm can be induced to stop for a short period of time—usually no more than two to four minutes—and that during this "still point" a person typically experiences a profound relief from chronic stress patterns. In fact, when the rhythm returns after a craniosacral still point, there is usually much more energy flowing through the nervous system and much better communication between different parts of the body. Especially when coupled with other techniques of craniosacral therapy, available from a skilled practitioner, many people report a phenomenal sense of ease and relaxation and clarity, and an almost unbelievable "spaciousness," especially in their heads and often in other parts of the body.

Not everyone has access to a skilled craniosacral practitioner. Fortunately, there is a way to induce a craniosacral stillpoint for yourself, anytime and almost anywhere. To do this, however, you'll need to track down and acquire some very sophisticated technology: two tennis balls and an old sock.

To make your craniosacral stillpoint inducer, put two tennis balls (actually, very dense foam rubber balls of the same size work a little better if you can find them) into either a sock or a cut length of sheer, stretch hosiery. The leg part of an old pair of panty hose will do nicely. You'll need to tie off the open ends so that the tennis balls don't move when pressure is put on them. The two balls should be touching when the sock is tied so that they won't form a gap between them later on when your head rests on them.

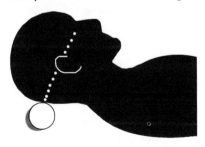

Using the craniosacral stillpoint inducer

To use the stillpoint inducer, lie down comfortably on your back on a firm surface—the floor, a massage table, or a firm bed. Slip the stillpoint inducer under your neck, with one ball on the left side and one on the right side, and then either scrunch yourself down or slip the stillpoint inducer up until it comes to rest under the bony, lower part of your skull. This is important: The stillpoint inducer must not be on your neck.

When it's correctly aligned, the center of the tennis balls will line up with the top of your ear (not the opening, but the top of the ear flaps). You should feel a space where the balls naturally rest against the occipital bone. If they're too low and touch your neck, they can cut off circulation and be quite painful. But when they're under the occipital bone, you should feel quite balanced and relaxed.

Usually, the stillpoint inducer should be kept in this position for between ten and twenty minutes. If you feel any discomfort, any headache sensations, you should stop immediately. A good position will, for most people, be very relaxing and after about five minutes can help promote a strong sense of calmness.

Although this technique is generally extremely safe, there are some people who should not use it for a variety of reasons. In general, a stillpoint inducer should not be used by:

- People who have ever had a stroke, aneurysm or cerebral hemorrhage. Skilled practitioners can adjust their touch to work effectively with these people but they should not use the mechanical device.

- People with osteoporosis, Down's syndrome, or others conditions associated with weakness of the vertebrae of the neck.

- Persons who have fractured their skulls or been treated for a rupture of the *dura mater* (the thick tissue under the skull that covers the brain) any time during the previous twelve months.

- Anyone who has had any epidural procedure during the previous six months.

- Children less than fourteen years since their cranial bones are still fairly soft. Again, a skilled practitioner can work effectively with young people but a mechanical device may be too rough for them.

- People who have recently experienced any unusual or recurring but undiagnosed dizziness, headaches, or abnormal vision.

- Anyone who has been diagnosed with any serious medical condition in which pressure changes in the skull could be dangerous, including brain tumors or hydrocephalic conditions ("water on the brain").

BIOFEEDBACK

Biofeedback training is designed to help people learn to use their minds to regulate body functions such as heart rate, blood pressure, muscle tension, and brain activity. Generally, sensitive monitoring devices are attached to the individual to measure and record a variety of physical responses such as skin temperature and electrical resistance, brain-wave activity, and respiration rate. These sensors monitor the body's physiological response to stress—for instance, muscle contraction during a tension headache—and then feed the information back using auditory and visual cues. By observing their own responses and following instructions given by highly trained biofeedback technicians, most people are able to exert some degree of conscious control over these body functions. Biofeedback is especially effective for helping people learn to manage stress, and it has become mainstream medical treatment for conditions such as high blood

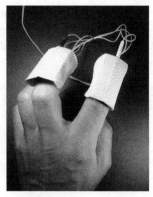

Biofeedback sensors

pressure, asthma, migraine headaches, hot flashes, and nausea associated with chemotherapy.

There is a wealth of clinical evidence about the efficacy of treatment of a variety of sleep disorders with biofeedback training, including sleep problems that may be attributable to developmental neurological problems, as well as for sleep problems most often observed in children, such as bedwetting, sleepwalking and sleep talking, night terrors, anxiety-related difficulties falling asleep, and insomnia. There also is promising evidence of the ability of the use of biofeedback to treat the most commons sleep problems of adults—insomnia and sleep apnea.

The National Institutes of Health (NIH) and the American Academy of Sleep Medicine consider biofeedback used in conjunction with relaxation training as potentially useful for helping to relieve sleep problems. In 1996, an NIH Technology Assessment Panel reviewed existing research and concluded that several non-pharmacological techniques, particularly relaxation and biofeedback, produced measurable improvements in some aspects of sleep, but questioned whether the improvements in sleep onset and total sleep time were large enough to be deemed clinically significant. Following their 1998 review of the relevant literature, the American Academy of Sleep Medicine recommended biofeedback along with progressive muscle relaxation for insomnia. The academy rated biofeedback as "probably efficacious"—the same rating given to cognitive-behavioral therapy for treatment of sleep disorders.

Yoga

Ayurvedic medicine (also called Ayurveda, which means "science of life") is believed to be the oldest medical tradition, and it has been practiced in India and Asia for more than five thousand years. With an emphasis on preventing disease and promoting wellness, its practitioners view emotional health and spiritual balance as vital for physical health and disease prevention. Ayurveda also considers diet, hygiene, sleep, lifestyle, and healthy relationships as powerful influences on health.

Practitioners aim to balance the three *doshas*—fundamental human qualities that they believe reside in varying concentrations in different parts of the human body. The doshas are thought to be disturbed by improper diet, sleep deprivation, travel, coffee, alcohol, or excessive exposure to the sun, and are balanced with diet, exercise, detoxification (ritual cleansing of toxins), yoga, spiritual counseling, herbal medicine, breathing exercises, and chanting.

One of the underlying principles of Ayurveda is that disease and disorders are caused by indigestion or failure to completely metabolize and integrate the foods, information, or experiences we take in. Using this perspective, Ayurveda might characterize sleep disorders or insomnia as a kind of mental or emotional indigestion—the inability to fully take in and then appropriately excrete the waste from, or in this case let go of, experiences, memories, traumas, or other problems. Mental indigestion might simply be the stress and overload of a busy day, the aftermath of an unpleasant encounter with a boss or coworker, or even the persistent mental energy we expend when we are deliberating about a problem in an effort to solve it. Emotional indigestion is the reappearance of an emotion—sadness, anger, or guilt—long after the experience or event that triggered the emotion.

Yogis (people who incorporate the practice of yoga in their lives) assert that yoga practice, which emphasizes self-awareness, balance, and self-regulation, benefits sleep in many ways. They opine that yoga improves the quality of sleep because of its stimulatory effect on the nervous system and the brain. Certain yoga postures increase the blood circulation to the sleep center in the brain and stimulate the parasympathetic nervous system, which promotes relaxation and acts to normalize the sleep cycle.

According to the NIH, regular yoga practice can help reduce anxiety, slow breathing, lower blood pressure, alter brain waves, and assist your heart to work more efficiently. Moreover, unlike aerobic or strenuous exercise or even vigorous yoga such as Ashtanga, which when practiced too close to bedtime may interfere with sleep, the deep rhythmic breathing and long, slow, gentle stretches of yoga may be practiced before bedtime. Many yoga poses (asanas) encourage both mind and body to slow, which promotes calm and sleep, and the extended exhale of yoga breathing creates an oxygen/carbon dioxide ratio in the bloodstream that is conducive to sleep.

There is even a designated "sleep yoga" practice. Tibetan sleep yoga is described as more than simply a practice for the night; it is a tool for awakening, which helps yogis integrate waking, sleeping and meditation with clear awareness. Proper position of the body and a calm mind are achieved using images

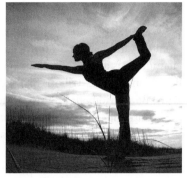

Practicing yoga can help promote relaxation and normalize the sleep cycle.

and visualizations as well as physical exercises. The overarching goal of sleep yoga practice is the pure experience of rigpa—the primordial, non-dual awareness advocated by the Dzogchen teachings—the luminous, open awareness that is the true nature of the mind.

Herbs and Dietary Supplements to Ease Stress and Promote Sleep

Along with a healthy, varied diet, regular exercise, and relaxation, many people find that herbs and dietary supplements offer stress-relief benefits—helping them to unwind, feel calm, and get restful, rejuvenating sleep. The following list is neither exhaustive nor complete—it is simply an overview of some naturally occurring herbs and supplements commonly used to relieve stress and promote sleep.

BREWER'S YEAST

Brewer's yeast (*Saccharomyces cerevisiae*) contains all the essential amino acids, fourteen minerals, and seventeen vitamins. It is a rich source of protein and of the B vitamins— B1 (thiamine), B2 (riboflavin), B3 (niacin), B5 (pantothenic acid), B6 (pyridoxine), B9 (folic acid), and H (biotin)— and other nutrients, such as selenium and chromium.

Many health professionals feel that supplementing B-complex vitamins is important during times of physical or emotional stress. It also delivers beta-glucans, which promote wound healing and the synthesis of RNA, an immune-enhancing nucleic acid that may help to prevent degenerative diseases and slow the aging process.

CHAMOMILE

Chamomile is a popular remedy for many ailments, including sleep disorders, anxiety, problems with digestion, skin infections, and inflammatory skin conditions such as eczema, as well as wound healing, infants' colic, teething pains, and diaper rash. Chamomile tea is known for its calming and mild sedating effects.

GINSENG

Ginseng (*Panax ginseng*) products are often called tonics, but the complementary and alternative medical literature has more aptly described them as adaptogens, because advocates of their use assert that ginseng increases resistance to physical, chemical, and biological stress and builds up vitality, including the physical and mental capacity for work.

Many users report that ginseng helps to reduce fatigue, boost energy, and promote physical endurance. The main active ingredients in ginseng are twenty-five complex carbohydrates called ginsenosides, some of which help to prevent excessive production of corticosteroids in response to physical, biological, or chemical stress.

Hops

Hops are the female flowers of *Humulus lupulus* L., a flowering vine native to North America, Asia, and Europe. They are traditionally used for relaxation, sedation, and to treat insomnia. Ancient Hebrews used hops to help ward off plague. In North America, several Native American tribes used hops as a sedative and sleep aid. Pillows filled with hops were used to sleep on, and hops have been used to flavor beer since the sixteenth century.

Hops are chemically complex and contain many different compounds. Researchers have identified several components that are sedative in nature, although it is not yet known whether hops contain enough of these compounds to actually cause sedation or drowsiness. Nonetheless, the German Federal Health Agency's Commission E has approved hops for sleep problems, restlessness, and anxiety. Research studies have considered hops in combination with valerian for the treatment of sleep disturbances, and several animal studies have examined the sedative properties of hops alone.

Most studies in humans have only tested the effects of hops on sleep quality when used in combination with valerian. Although this research does suggest effectiveness, most studies have been inconclusive and in many trials, the effects of hops cannot be distinguished from the benefits of valerian.

KAVA

Kava (*Piper methysticum*) is an herbal remedy used to ease symptoms of stress, anxiety, and depression. Its primary active ingredients are kavalactones, compounds that may produce mild sedation and muscle relaxation and reduce anxiety. It also has been found to improve mood, cognitive performance, and quality of sleep. Several rigorous clinical trials demonstrated kava's efficacy in the treatment of anxiety, and some preliminary evidence indicates that it may be as effective as the benzodiazepine drugs—such as alprazolam (Xanax), chlordiazepoxide (Librium), diazepam (Valium), and lorazepam (Ativan)—in terms of relieving anxiety. Several cases of liver damage from kava use have been reported. Consult with your medical practitioner before using kava if you have liver disease or other serious medical conditions.

LEMON BALM

Lemon balm (*Melissa officinalis*) is a lemon-scented member of the mint family that has a mildly sedating effect. It has been used since the Middle Ages to reduce stress and anxiety, promote sleep, improve appetite, and ease pain and discomfort associated with digestive disorders. One study of people with minor sleep disorders who took a combination of valerian and lemon balm reported sleeping much better than those who were given placebo.

L-THEANINE

L-theanine is a non-protein amino acid that occurs naturally in the green tea plant (*Camellia sinensis*). L-theanine makes up 50 percent of the total free amino acids in the green tea plant. It gives green tea its distinctive aroma and flavor. Historically,

L-theanine has been used as a relaxing agent and in Japan, L-theanine is widely used as a nutritional supplement for to influence mood. Although its mechanism of action has not yet been fully described, it may affect the metabolism and the release of some neurotransmitters in the brain. Its ability to induce relaxation may be attributable to its effects on serotonin, dopamine, and other neurotransmitters.

PASSION FLOWER

Passion flower is a sweet delicious fruit that is eaten raw or cooked in jellies. Its leaves are served as a cooked vegetable or eaten raw in salads. Recent research indicated that the bioflavonoids in passion flower are very likely responsible for its observed relaxing and anti-anxiety effects. Many homeopathic remedies contain passion flower; it is possible that the plant's mechanism of action is homeopathic.

When Spanish explorers first encountered passion flower plants in Peru and Brazil, they found it was used in native folk medicine as a sedative. Its use gradually spread throughout Europe, where it was used as a sedative and to induce sleep.

Today, more than four hundred species of passion flower are found throughout the world. Modern day research reveals that passion flower produces a mild sedative effect that encourages sleep. Researchers have documented that it appears to reduce nervous symptoms and cramps that inhibit sleep, and promote restful, uninterrupted, deep sleep. Since many recent studies have tested products that combine other ingredients with passion flower, it is not yet known if alone it can be recommended for the treatment of restlessness, anxiety, or insomnia.

RHODIOLA ROSEA

Rhodiola rosea has been used to combat fatigue, enhance mental clarity, speed recovery from illness, prevent infections, and enhance sexual function. Because it is an adaptogen, it helps the body adjust to physical and psychological stress and helps to return the body to balance and equilibrium. Its adaptogenic effects and central nervous system activities are primarily due to its ability to influence both the levels and activity of serotonin, dopamine, and norepinephrine in the cerebral cortex, brain stem, and hypothalamus.

Rhodiola rosea has been shown to prevent catecholamine release and subsequent cyclic AMP elevation in the myocardium (heart muscle), and the depletion of adrenal catecholamines induced by acute stress. A double-blind, placebo-controlled study looking at use of rhodiola extract among male military cadets suffering from sleep deprivation and stress found that rhodiola was more effective than placebo at fighting the effects of stress and fatigue.

VALERIAN

Valerian (*Valeriana officinalis*) has been used as a sedative and to relieve anxiety and insomnia for more than two thousand years. Although it contains many bioactive compounds, valerian's sedative and hypnotic properties are attributed to sesquiterpenes of the volatile oil.

Clinical studies have demonstrated that it is more effective than placebo at improving the duration and quality of sleep among persons suffering from insomnia. It has also proven effective as an anxiolytic (having anti-anxiety action)—and several randomized controlled studies found it more effective than placebo at relieving physiological measures of stress, such as blood pressure and heart rate, as well as subjects' self-reported feelings of stress.

SKULLCAP

Skullcap (*Scutellaria lateriflora*) comes from the mint family and traditionally has been used as a nerve tonic and mild sedative to relieve anxiety, nerve pain, muscle spasms, headaches, exhaustion, and insomnia. Its bioactive compounds are wogonin and baicalin, flavonoids thought to promote mild relaxation and affect the nervous and musculoskeletal systems.

TYROSINE

Tyrosine is a nonessential amino acid that is synthesized in the body from phenylalanine. It is needed to make epinephrine, norepinephrine, serotonin, and dopamine, all of which work to regulate mood. Deficiencies in tyrosine have been linked to depression. Tyrosine plays a key role in the manufacture and regulation of adrenal, thyroid, and pituitary gland hormones and is involved in the synthesis of encephalin, which is the name of two substances that are used as neurotransmitters, and, because they are natural opiates, act as sedatives and analgesics.

MELATONIN

Melatonin is a neurohormone produced in the brain by the pineal gland, from the amino acid tryptophan. Its synthesis and release are stimulated by darkness and suppressed by light, indicating that it plays an important role in the circadian rhythm. Blood levels of melatonin are highest just before bedtime. Melatonin supplements have been used to help travelers recover from jet lag and to treat insomnia and other sleep disorders.

Because melatonin use is so popular among people suffering from sleep disorders, NCCAM funded research that analyzed available scientific evidence supporting its safety, efficacy, and known risks. The researchers found that melatonin seems safe for short-term use but may not be effective for treating sleep disorders such as jet lag. On the other hand, it shows promise for delayed sleep phase syndrome. Melatonin's precise mechanism of action has not yet been uncovered and further research is needed to determine its best use in treating sleep disorders.

5-HTP: THE SERENITY OF SEROTONIN

As we've seen, the brain and nervous system are deeply involved in every aspect of human life, including our responses to stress and the sleep/wake cycle. While nerve cells talk to one another using electrical impulses, neurotransmitters shape and direct their communication by amplifying, relaying, blocking or modulating a wide variety of nervous system messages.

Serotonin is one of the most important of these neurotransmitters and has been identified as a key regulator of mood, sleep, sexuality, and appetite. Many antidepressant drugs work by blocking the body's reabsorption of serotonin, effectively keeping each molecule in play for a longer period of time. These SSRIs—selective serotonin reuptake inhibitors—include drugs like Prozac, Zoloft, and Paxil.

It's tempting to think that we can help to relieve our stress, anxiety, or depression by taking extra serotonin in the form of a pill or potion. Unfortunately, the serotonin molecule doesn't pass through the protective barrier between the bloodstream and the brain. Any serotonin we consume directly will simply be broken down without doing any us good. In fact, the venom of stinging insects like bees and wasps actually contains serotonin. When injected under the skin, serotonin acts as a painful irritant!

The body's level of serotonin can, however, be influenced by consuming the nutritional precursors from which the body makes serotonin. Serotonin is synthesized from the amino acid tryptophan, which is then converted into an intermediate chemical form called 5-hydroxytryptophan, or 5-HTP for short. Many people report that taking 5-HTP brightens their mood, improves the quality of sleep, helps them to resist depression and anxiety, and relieves many symptoms of stress.

In the body, 5-HTP passes through the blood-brain barrier where it is converted into serotonin (whose chemical name is 5-hydroxytryptamine, abbreviated 5-HT). While this nutritional approach works well for a great many people, the relationships between neurotransmitter levels, mood, and behavior are very complex and highly individual.

Now, blessings light on him that first invented sleep! It covers a man all over, thoughts and all, like a cloak; it is meat for the hungry, drink for the thirsty, heat for the cold, and cold for the hot. It is the current coin that purchases all the pleasures of the world cheap, and the balance that sets the king and the shepherd, the fool and the wise man, even.

—Miguel de Cervantes, *Don Quixote*, 1605

References

N. Ayas, et al. "A Prospective Study of Sleep Duration and Coronary Heart Disease in Women." *Arch Intern Med.* 2003; 163(2):205–09.

C.P. Cannon, C.H. McCabe, P.H. Stone, et al. "Circadian Variation in the Onset of Unstable Angina and Non-Q-wave acute Myocardial Infarction (the TIMI III Registry and TIMI IIIB)." *American Journal of Cardiology.* 1997; 79(3): 253–58.

P.K. Capp, et al. "Pediatric Sleep Disorders." *Prim Care Clin Office Pract.* 2005; 32:549–62.

M.A. Carskadon, C. Acebo, G.S. Richardson, B.A.Tate, and R. Seifer. "An Approach to Studying Circadian Rhythms of Adolescent Humans." *Journal of Biological Rhythms.* 1997; 12: 278–89.

G. Copinschi. "Metabolic and Endocrine Effects of Sleep Deprivation." *Essent Psychopharmacol.* 2005; 6(6):341–47.

B.H. Fox, J.S. Robbin. "The Retention of Material Presented During Sleep." *Journal of Experimental Psychology,* 1952; 43:75–79.

"French Health Minister Seeks Nap Study." Associated Press. January 31, 2007.

J.E. Gangwisch, et al. "Short Sleep Duration as a Risk Factor for Hypertension: Analyses of the First National Health and Nutrition Examination Survey." *Hypertension.* 2006; 47(5):833–39.

D.R. Gold, et al. "Rotating Shift Work, Sleep, and Accidents Related to Sleepiness in Hospital Nurses." *Am J Public Health*.1992; 82:1011–14.

I.S. Hairston, et al. "Sleep Restriction Suppresses Neurogenesis Induced by Hippocampus-dependent Learning." *J Neurophysiol.* 2005; 94(6):4224–33.

J.C. Hall. "Cryptochromes: Sensory Reception, Transduction, and Clock Functions Subserving Circadian Systems." *Current Opinion in Neurobiology.* 2000; 10(4): 456–66.

E. Hartmann. "Why Do We Dream?" ScientificAmerican.com. July 10, 2006. http://sciam/askexpert_question.cfm?articleID =00072867-D925-1F0E-97AE80A84189EEDF, accessed Febru–ary 16, 2007.

D. Healy, M.A. Runco. "Could Creativity Be Associated With Insomnia?" *Creativity Research Journal,* 2006; 18(1):39–43.

"Insomnia: Assessment and Management in Primary Care." National Center on Sleep Disorders Research and Office of Prevention, Education and Control, National Institutes of Health National Heart, Lung, and Blood Institute. Bethesda, MD, 1998.

M.R. Irwin. "Sleep deprivation and activation of morning levels of cellular and genomic markers of inflammation." *Arch Intern Med.* 2006; 166(16):1756–62.

N.N. Jarjour. "Circadian Variation in Allergen and Nonspecific Bronchial Responsiveness in Asthma." *Chronobiology International.* 1999; 16(5): 631–39.

W.D.S. Kilgore, et al. "The effects of 53 hours of sleep deprivation on moral judgment." *Sleep.* 2007; 30(3):345–52.

L. Lamber. "Familial Link *Seen* in Obstructive Sleep Apnea." *Journal of the American Medical Association.* 2003; 290(22): 2925–26.

L. Lamberg. "Experts Study Consequences of Sleep Deprivation." *Psychiatric News.* 2002;37(16):20.

D. Léger, et al. "Allergic Rhinitis and Its Consequences on Quality of Sleep: An Unexplored Area." *Arch Intern Med.* 2006;166(16):1744–48.

E. Leibenluft, P.S. Albert, N.E. Rosenthal, et al. "Relationship between Sleep and Mood in Patients with Rapid-cycling Bipolar Disorder." *Psychiatry Research.* 1996; 63(2–3): 161–68.

J. Marin, et al. "Long-term Cardiovascular Outcomes in Men with Obstructive Sleep Apnoea-hypopnoea with or without Treatment with Continuous Positive Airway Pressure: An Observational Study." *Lancet.* 2005;365(9464):1046–53.

D. Markov, M. Goldman. "Normal Sleep and Circadian Rhythms: Neurobiological Mechanisms Underlying Sleep and Wakefulness." *Psychiatr Clin N Am.* 2006; 29:841–53.

L.J. Meltzer, J.A. Mindell. "Sleep and Sleep Disorders in Children and Adolescents." *Psychiatr Clin N Am.* 2006; 1059–76.

"Narcolepsy Fact Sheet." National Institute of Neurological Disorders and Stroke. National Institutes of Health, Bethesda, MD, 2007. http://www.ninds.nih.gov/disorders/narcolepsy/detail_narcolepsy.htm, accessed March 9, 2007.

A. Naska, et al. "Siesta in Healthy Adults and Coronary Mortality in the General Population." *Arch Intern Med.* 2007; 167:296–301.

National Heart, Lung, and Blood Institute. 1998. "Insomnia: assessment and management in primary care" (NIH Pub. No. 98–4088). Bethesda, MD: NHLBI.

"Nonpsychotropic Drugs May Cause Sleep Disturbances." *Drug Ther Perspect.* 1997; 10(12):10–13.

N.J. Pearson, et al. "Insomnia, Trouble Sleeping, and Complementary and Alternative Medicine: Analysis of the 2002 National Health Interview Survey Data." *Arch Intern Med.* 2006; 166(16):1775–82.

P.D. Penev. "Association Between Sleep and Morning Testosterone Levels in Older Men." *Sleep.* 2007; 30(4):427–32.

P.E. Peppard, et al. "Longitudinal Association of Sleep-Related Breathing Disorder and Depression." *Arch Intern Med.* 2006; 166(16):1709–15.

G.E. Pickard, F.W. Turek. "The Suprachiasmatic Nuclei: Two Circadian Clocks?" *Brain Research.* 1983; 268(2): 201–10.

A. Rechtschaffen. "Current Perspectives on the Function of Sleep." *Perspectives in Biological Medicine*, 1998; 41: 359–90.

K.J. Reid, H.J. Burgess. "Circadian Rhythm Sleep Disorders." *Prim Care Clin Office Pract.* 2005; 32:449–73.

T. Rozhon. "To Have, Hold and Cherish, Until Bedtime." *New York Times.* March 11, 2007.

N. Singer. "Hey, Sleepy, Want to Buy a Good Nap?" *New York Times.* February 1, 2007.

K. Spiegel, R. Leproult, E. Van Cauter. "Impact of Sleep Debt on Metabolic and Endocrine Function." *Lancet.* 1999; 354:1435–39.

K. Spiegel, J.F. Sheridan, E.Van Cauter. "Effect of Sleep Deprivation on Response to Immunization." *JAMA.* 2002; 288:1471–72.

"Subcommittee on Railroads, Pipelines, and Hazardous Materials—Fatigue in the Rail Industry." February 13, 2007. http://transportation.house.gov/hearings/hearingdetail/aspx ?NewsID=29, accessed April 1, 2007.

H.P.A. Van Dongen, et al. "The Cumulative Cost of Additional Wakefulness: Dose-response Effects on Neurobehavioral Functions and Sleep Physiology from Chronic Sleep Restriction and Total Sleep Deprivation." *Sleep.* 2003; 26:117–26.

G. Vazquez-Palacios, et al. "Copulatory Activity Increases Slow-wave Sleep in the Male Rat." *Journal of Sleep Research.* 2002; 11(3):237–45.

R. von Kanel, et al. "Association Between Polysomnographic Measures of Disrupted Sleep and Prothrombotic Factors." *Chest.* 2007; 131(3):733–39.

M.P. Walker, R. Stickgold, D. Alsop, N. Gaab, G. Schlaug. "Sleep-dependent Motor Memory Plasticity in the Human Brain." *Neuroscience.* 2005; 133(4):911–17.

P.C. Zee, F.W. Turek. "Sleep and Health: Everywhere and in Both Directions." *Arch Intern Med.* 2006; 166(16):1686–88.

Index